THE GOLDEN SECRETS TO OPTIMAL HEALTH

THE GOLDEN SECRETS TO OPTIMAL HEALTH

Revealing a holistic, unconventional guide to feeling and looking your best—for you, your family and the environment.

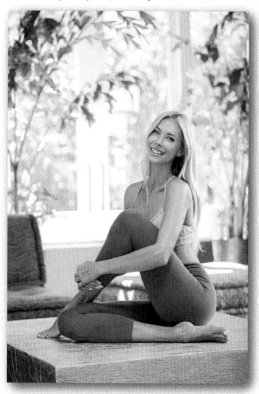

Jesse Golden

Dedication

I dedicate this book to all the people who have inspired me, motivated me, and questioned the things we are told about health.

To all the people who have a desire to live a longer, healthier, happier life so that they can serve and share their light, because without them, I would never have found my path toward optimal health.

Having rheumatoid arthritis drove me to discover my passion for empowering myself and others to live healthy lives, and it taught me that there is not just one way to cure disease. Rather "dis-ease" starts in the mind, and the mind has to be clear to make wise choices. I believe sickness is given to us to discover this.

Wisdom Prevention Vitality

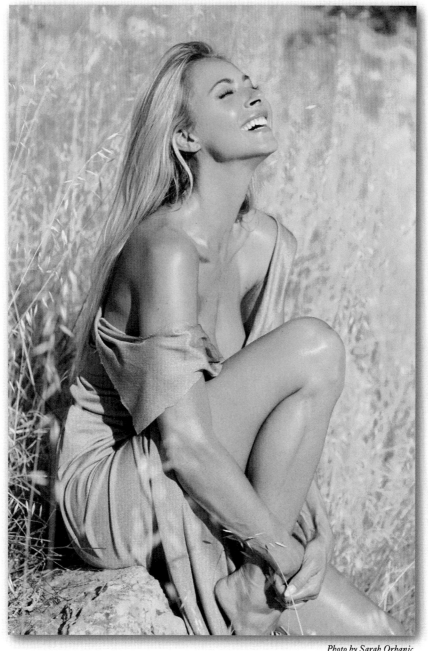

I mprove your quality of life and state of mind, increase your strength and mobility, optimize your weight, extend your warranty, and tap into the fountain of youth.

Contents

Foreword

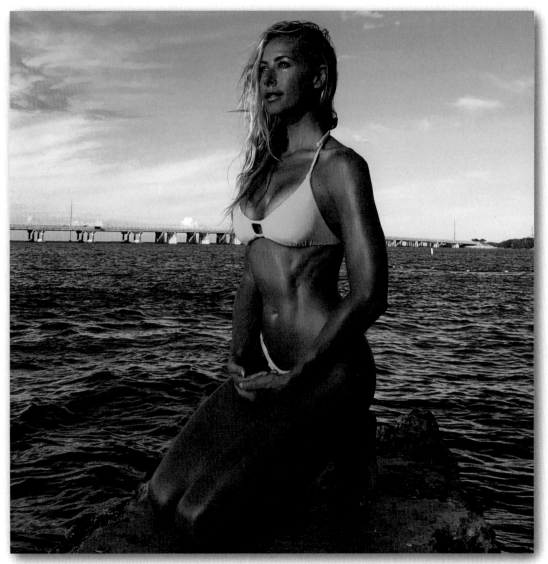

Photo by Maryann Golden

Whether you suffer from a chronic or acute disease, or you are currently as "healthy as a horse," you need to take responsibility for what you can do to prevent illness and protect yourself, your family, and the environment. Doctors are not responsible for your health; you are!

When you get sick, I believe you are at a crossroad; either you are going to make positive changes or you are going to remain sick.

With all the artificial and genetically modified foods produced today and our unnatural and toxic environments, our dietary and spiritual needs have changed and will continue to do so.

Every day there seems to be a new chronic disease or virus that spreads, knocking everyone down in its path. Every single one of us knows at least one person who has been affected by cancer, for example. It is up to us to change this! We need to make positive, conscious, mindful choices every day. Not only for ourselves but for the "whole." Understanding that, we are not separate. All of us are connected to each other and the environment, and every positive frequency we send out into the world raises the vibration of the whole planet.

What affects one of us will eventually affect all of us. This is not new wisdom. It is ancient knowledge that we need to remember and return to.

We're all in this together. Let's manifest a health revolution!

> *The process of self-healing is the privilege of every being. Self-healing is not a miracle, nor is self-healing a dramatization of the personality as though you could do something superior. Self-healing is a genuine process of the relationship between the physical and the infinite power of the soul.*
>
> —*YOGI BHAJAN*

Acknowledgments

My son Kaleo, who is my angel sent from heaven, my greatest teacher, inspiration, love, and light.

My mother, who showed me that women can be dynamic, who always supported me in my unconventional ways of being, and who loved me unconditionally.

My grandmother, who taught me that everything can be fixed with a good song, a good laugh, and a glass of B&B.

My dad, for showing me firsthand how the power of a positive mind and kind heart can heal and overcome.

My Aunt Dianne, for always being my sounding board and sharing her love and wisdom.

My best friends (you know who you are): thank you for your unwavering love and support.

My cousin Jessica, who lit the way and without whom I would not be who I am today.

Deb, for your Knowingness always talking truth to my Knowingness.

Sarah, for your devoted contribution to most of the photos taken in this book (including the covers) and your exquisite ability to capture one's true essence.

To all the photographers whose work is in this book; I have such admiration and gratitude for your skill. Every image tells a story and exudes a feeling that inspires my message.

And, of course, my tribe, my siStars, my followers and fans, who have motivated and inspired me to share my story—this is for you!

My Story

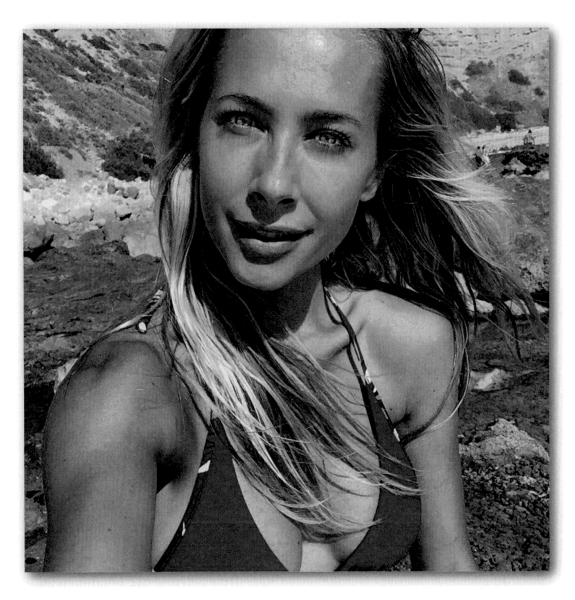

I grew up in Chicago, Illinois, in the 1980s and 1990s, when microwaves, fast food, and canned vegetables were all the rage. I grew up drinking soda pop and eating deep-dish pizza and beef sandwiches. At age eleven I got food poisoning from eating undercooked meat. At that time, a fad in the Midwest was restaurants where you picked out your own raw meat from huge refrigerators and you cooked it on large family-style grills. Well, I didn't cook my meat thoroughly enough, and that night, I literally dreamt of cows mooing and mooing, and I woke up very ill.

I believe that was the first time I made the connection between food and its effect on my body.

In that moment I told my mom I was never going to eat meat again. I joined the organization People for the Ethical Treatment of Animals (PETA) and tried to get everyone I knew on the bandwagon of vegetarianism. I became very vocal about my beliefs on this subject, and my family considered this to be "abnormal" behavior.

I remember my grandmother saying to me, "You are going to die if you don't eat meat."

Well, I didn't die, and I am grateful that my mom honored my decision and took me to a nutritionist to help me with supplementing protein and iron in my diet. For the first time, I was introduced to tofu, the value of beans and lentils, and a variety of vegetables that I had never heard of before. I remained a vegetarian and activist until I was twenty-one, and then…I started craving meat. Most likely due to not eating properly.

In addition to the fear of how my body would react, I was embarrassed and humiliated just thinking about having to reverse the stance I had been taking for ten years by telling everyone I was no longer a vegetarian. After much contemplation, soul-searching, and ignoring my primal instincts multiple times, I finally gave in.

I remember this surrender being a very ceremonial experience for me. I was away on a modeling job and I ordered room service…chicken breast, very well done! I sat there on the bed in the hotel, all alone, staring at my chicken. I said a prayer and took one bite and then waited, as I thought my body might internally combust. Slowly, I took bite after bite and was able to eat the entire meal, and, to my surprise, I felt good!

From that point on, I began reexploring foods that I had not eaten in years. Looking back at that time, I ate everything and anything I wanted, but I still found myself preferring a more pesco-vegetarian diet. It was nice to just have the freedom to try foods and not have to ask what was in it all the time. I had an enormous appetite, but continued to stay fit through my active lifestyle.

Then at twenty-five years young, I became pregnant and indulged even more in the food I wanted. As many women do, I felt like I couldn't deny the baby (ha-ha). At nine months pregnant, I weighed 185 pounds and intended to have a natural birth. My midwife said if I wanted to have a natural childbirth, I had better slow down on my food intake. I increased my walking and Kundalini yoga practice, slowed down on all the sweet cravings, and was able to have a natural home water birth. My beautiful son, Kaleo Golden, weighed a plump and healthy eight pounds. Right after his birth, I realized that much of my weight was water. I breastfed my son for four years and was always very active, so the weight naturally came off.

When Kaleo was four years young, I started to notice that my body was showing signs that something was wrong. As a single mother still breastfeeding, I always had an excuse for why I was tired, sore, or not feeling well. But the symptoms progressed, so I went to my doctor for a checkup. After being misdiagnosed, and then jumping from doctor to doctor, I was finally diagnosed with rheumatoid arthritis, a disheartening realization.

Scared, desperate, and feeling defeated, I started the treatment my doctor prescribed, as I was told the quicker and more aggressively the disease was treated, the more likely it would go into remission. I was given a combination therapy of disease-modifying anti-rheumatic drugs (DMARDS), including methotrexate, which is a chemotherapy agent and immunosuppressant. This was the first time my body had any pharmaceuticals or medicine in years. I had never been one to even take an over-the-counter drug for a minor ailment. I preferred and always relied on natural modalities. So naturally, I researched what I could do through my diet.

I went back to being a vegetarian, a lifestyle I was familiar with, and I learned additional information about inflammation-triggering foods, such as nightshades and gluten. I created a diet that I thought was suitable for healing my body, but due to my illness and new medications, I lacked energy and motivation; it was all I could do to make sure my son was well fed and taken care of, let alone having to create new recipes for myself. I also had a fear that everything I ate would cause me more pain, and what ended up happening is that I did not eat enough food to sustain my body.

Within days of starting my prescribed treatment plan, I began to experience several severe adverse reactions—reactions that began to overshadow my original diagnosis. In the back of my mind I knew that my body would reject such treatment, but in my vulnerable state I wanted to believe that it could help. Looking back, it was all part of the process, and it gave me the motivation and drive I needed to dedicate myself to Eastern medicine.

Through a dear friend I was introduced to a macrobiotic counselor. After being diagnosed twenty-five years prior with stage four cancer, this counselor had been given a couple months to live and she was now well. Through the macrobiotic lifestyle, she had become a walking legend with a long list of clients that had chronic diseases and were cured holistically.

I was excited to start this path, and with the support of my family and friends, I dove in 100 percent. It literally "took a village" to do what was required for this healing diet and to turn my body from acid to alkaline. I had a macrobiotic chef seven days a week. I stocked up on groceries every other day. I did tinctures, scrubs, baths, shiatsu treatments…everything I was aware of in order to lead me to wellness.

My entire life was timed—when I should eat, sleep, and walk, as well as when to do all my various healing practices. My diet consisted of fresh vegetables, sea vegetables, and grains. I ate no meat, except for one piece of fish (cod) per week, and no sugar, except for one baked apple per week. Everything I put into my body had a purpose to cleanse and heal.

However, when one's body is healing, it discharges and goes through something called a "healing crisis." I got very sick with fevers, a discharge of black mucus, bleeding gums, and more aches and pains—and of course, there was a tincture for the healing crisis too, so with the hope that once I got through this crisis, I would be healed, I carried on.

In the macrobiotic philosophy, it is believed that it takes ninety days for one's body to go from acid to alkaline, so I decided I was going to eat a macrobiotic diet for at least four months to see how my body responded.

Even though I was eating more than I had ever eaten before, the food was so wholesome and my body was so "clean" that the fat just melted off my body, and I didn't have much fat in the first place. Unable to work out, I lost all muscle tone and I weighed ninety pounds. At five feet, ten inches tall, that looks very scary.

On a spiritual level, I had never felt so clear: my brain was sharper than ever, my eyes were as white as they could be, and my skin even glowed. Yet after several months and thousands of dollars later, my health continued to decline and that light at the end of the tunnel seemed to disappear. My family intervened and begged me to go back to my rheumatologist. I thought perhaps they were right.

I knew in my heart that I had to try everything holistic and within my power before I would go back to Western medicine, and a year after my diagnosis, I could honestly say that I had tried everything. My quality of life had suffered, and most of all I felt like I was missing parts of motherhood that I would never get back. My reason for trying to heal myself was to be able to be there for my son, but it got to the point where it would have been selfish for me to go on any longer that way.

With my tail between my legs, I shuffled like an old lady into my doctor's office. She was astonished that I had let myself get to this state of ill health, and without taking even an ibuprofen. With limited options left, I decided to remain optimistic about her health suggestions. As I suspected, she wanted to start treatment right then and there, hooking me up to a steroids IV for an hour in order to bring down the inflammation I had in every synovial joint and organ in my body.

The other part of my treatment would consist of at-home shots of TNF blockers (immunosuppressants) every two weeks, with checkups and blood work every eight weeks, to make sure the medicine's side effects were not doing more damage than good.

Initially my body responded very well to the treatment suggested by my doctors. I believe it was because my system was so clean and I was forced to do the "inside work," putting me in a different mind frame. For the first time in a year, I had no pain and I could walk. In fact, I started running for the first time in my life. I was so grateful to be able to move again, and I was motivated to get into the best shape of my life and regain all the muscle mass I had lost. I continued with my macrobiotic diet, and since I was feeling better, I gave myself more freedom with food choices when dining out and being social.

Most rheumatoid arthritis patients have difficulty experiencing any relief, let alone remission or no signs of inflammation. I believe it was not just my diet or medication that caused my remission, but it was also my spiritual journey of learning about myself and listening to my "Knowingness." The symptoms of my disease were there to be my teacher, and until I learned what they were there to teach me, they remained in residence.

At this point in my journey, I had explored both Eastern and Western medicine, and I was determined to find a balance in which I could thrive. After a while, the side effects of my medication seemed to take over the symptoms of my disease again. After everything I had been through, I felt confident that I knew my body's triggers well enough to be able to go off all medication. I had my "toolbox" of remedies that I used when a symptom or issue pertaining to my disease would arise.

Under my doctor's care and with my unwavering decision, I weaned myself off the medication. There was an expected adjustment period, but I remained positive and steadfast in my goal.

I choose to thrive despite my diagnosis of rheumatoid arthritis.

I choose to look at rheumatoid arthritis as a blessing and not a curse. The disease has taught me and continues to teach me every day: about my limits, my compassion, my desires, and my spirituality. I am grateful for the days that I feel strong and for my continued lessons on days when I don't feel strong. My journey is not yet over. I realize that it will continue with twists and turns, and I am learning to adapt and be open to new ideas.

I don't believe that there is one pill, one diet, or one trick to cure my rheumatoid arthritis rather that it will the continuing effort to ride the wave with a positive and fluid mind that will keep me in remission.

It is listening to my Knowingness and letting it guide my way.

It is reversing my negative mental patterns that I have accepted along the way and healing internally by replacing these negative patterns with positive patterns.

Stay true to your body temple. There is not one remedy for all. We each must find our own path to optimum health.

—Jesse Golden

A wish written down becomes a goal. A goal backed by action becomes reality.
Write down the goals that you want to achieve in your health and life. Don't second-guess yourself. Just write what comes to mind.

_____

_____

_____

_____

_____

_____

_____

_____

_____

_____

_____

_____

#BeGolden

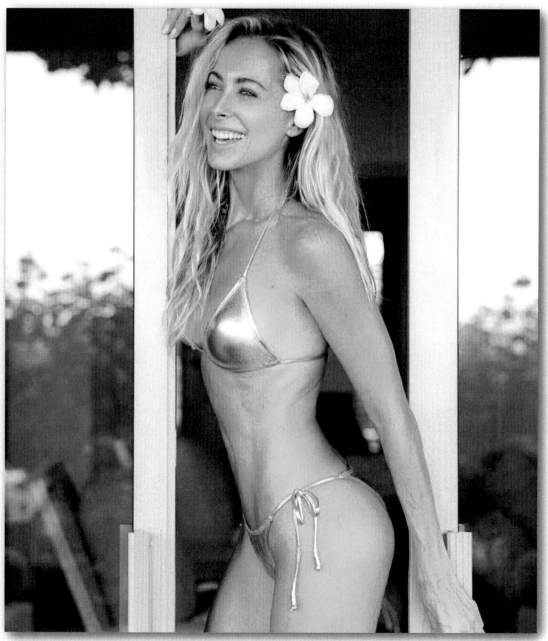

Photo by Sarah Orbanic

"Be Golden" means to be the best version of you! Flaws, ailments, imperfections, and all. To embrace who you are, and with that be successful, prosperous, thriving, radiant, and superb.

Your story is the key that could unlock someone else's prison. Share your light by sharing your testimonial.

Follow us on Instagram @*thegoldensecrets* and share your experience by posting about your journey. Inspire and support each other along the way! You never know whom you could be helping in a time of need.

> *The ability to heal yourself is far greater than anybody has given you permission to believe. I have been there and can testify to that fact.*
>
> —JESSE GOLDEN

Inspiration

In the midst of battling rheumatoid arthritis, at five feet, ten inches tall, I was less than ninety-five pounds. For months I was completely immobile, unable to walk or take care of myself. I lost all muscle tone, flexibility, strength, and half of my hair. Every joint and organ in my body was inflamed, and I was in constant pain, as if every bone in my body was broken.

This was the experience that changed my life. Not being able to move, I was forced to look internally and my medicine became a spiritual practice of dissolving the mental cause of rheumatoid arthritis, connecting my physical wounds to spiritual wounds that I had experienced in my life. These negative experiences created negative thought patterns that were creating my health issues. By replacing these negative patterns with positive ones, I was able to create a new, healthier experience for myself and begin to heal. I believe that for every physical condition, there is a mental cause associated with it.

> *If you don't listen to your body's signals, the signals will magnify until you have no choice but to listen.*

—JESSE GOLDEN

To the right are pictures of me during the many different phases of my life. Battling rheumatoid arthritis and the many side effects of both the disease and the medications. Pregnant with my son, Kaleo, I weighed 185 pounds. Yes, it was pregnancy weight, but I gained sixty-five pounds, which is higher than average for a single-baby pregnancy. Six months after giving birth with my son Kaleo. Thanks to breastfeeding and lots of walking, I was back to my normal weight and feeling great. Three years later I was diagnosed with rheumatoid arthritis.

I have experienced many health states in my life, from achieving ballerina status in my adolescence, symbolizing the epitome of health, to being completely disabled, unable to walk or physically care for myself. Through my story, I hope to inspire you and yours.

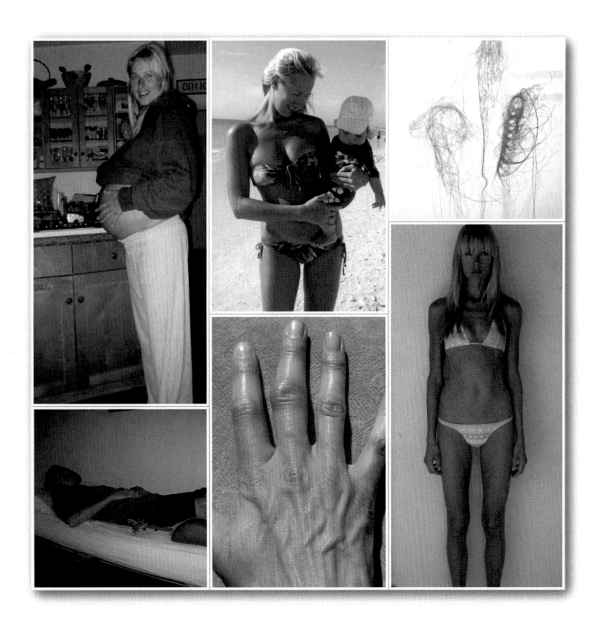

Below are pictures of the work I did after my rheumatoid arthritis went into remission. Every picture represents something I thought I might never be able to do again after I was diagnosed.

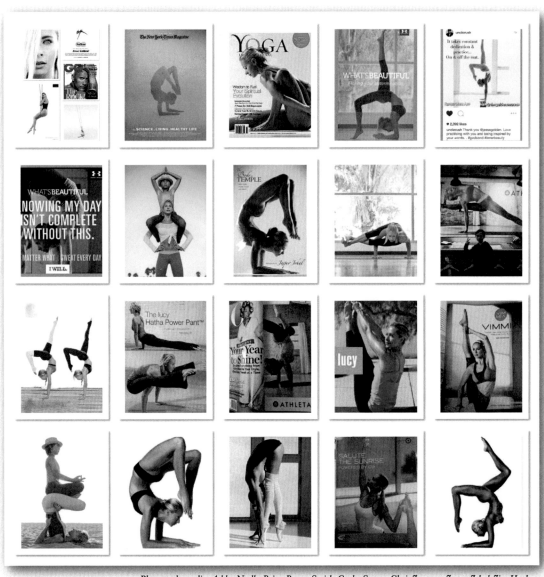

Photography credits: *Ashley Noelle, Brian Bowen Smith, Carlos Serrao, Chris Jameson, Jasper Johal, Jim Henken, Luke Wooden, Marcel Indik, Martin Rusch, Sarah Orbanic, Sophi Pangrazzi, Todd Cole, Todd Vitti*

Rheumatoid Arthritis Statistics

Rheumatoid arthritis is a chronic inflammatory disease that manifests itself in multiple joints of the body and can also affect the organs. According to the Center for Disease Control (www.cdc.gov):

- Rheumatoid arthritis (RA) causes premature death, disability, and lowers the quality of life of people in the industrialized and developing world.

- People with RA may experience more losses in function than people without arthritis in every domain of human activity including work, leisure, and social relations.

- In 2005 rheumatoid arthritis affected over 1.5 million Americans eighteen years of age and over.

- The specific cause of rheumatoid arthritis is not known, and there is no known cure for the disease.

Introduction

First of all, I want to say congratulations for making steps toward your optimal health and thank you for choosing my book. You are the reason I wrote it.

I am a holistic health practitioner, but most of my knowledge comes from my life experiences. My health challenges became blessings as I gained more knowledge than any textbook could have taught me and as I gained compassion for the human body and its ability to heal. Realizing that almost anything can be healed by our own lifestyle choices, my passion became to inspire you through my journey, in hopes that it would give you the courage and faith that you, too, can attain optimal health.

I am going to share with you the modalities that have worked for me and some things that didn't. Some of the things that worked for me will not be right for you, but I want to encourage you to seek and explore different options to find out what works for you.

No matter where you are in your life, your body, or your state of health, know that you are on the right path. The very fact that you are reading this tells me so. Through consistency and sincerity you can succeed.

THINGS TO KEEP IN MIND BEFORE STARTING YOUR JOURNEY:
Making time for yourself is the first step. Let go of guilt that you are taking time away from work or family. Trust me, if you follow my steps you will have increased energy and be more productive, thus affording you more time to be with the loved ones in your life. You will also be setting a good example for the people you care most about.

Don't abruptly change your life. Go at your own pace. This is not a competition. The challenge is for you to become a healthier, stronger, wiser version of you! That process looks different for everyone so don't compare yourself to what others are doing and instead take this time to focus on awakening parts of yourself you didn't know existed—slowly evolving and organically developing your willpower.

Focus on healthy, mindful choices every step of the way and your body will follow your lead. I always tell my students we are planting seeds. These seeds will blossom into flowers, but that process takes time. It is said that for every year of "dis-ease," it will take at least one month of natural health approaches to nurture you back to health.

Only you can make the positive changes needed to feel your absolute best. This occurs in your everyday routine and outside your comfort zone. Promise yourself that you will step outside of your comfort zone and explore different ideas and be open to change. This is how you grow. If the changes don't challenge you, then they don't change you.

Disease and health are both the result of the interaction of three aspects: body, mind, and spirit. Whatever we can do for our health ourselves is better than what others can.

LET'S BUILD A HEALTHY LIFESTYLE TOGETHER!

> *Change leads to disappointment if it is not sustained. Transformation is sustained change, and it is achieved through practice.*

> —*B. K. S. IYENGAR*

Be patient and kind to yourself through this journey to optimal health. The emotions, challenges, and triumphs will come in waves. Acknowledge them and know that they will pass. You are coming into your own.

Part 1
Nourish

Eat Right for You

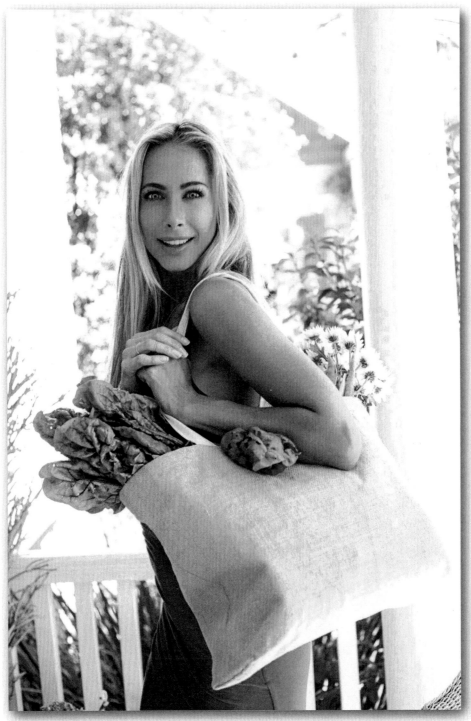

Photo by Ashley Noelle

Americans spend trillions of dollars every year on medical care to treat diseases, when the prevention of those diseases can be as simple as a change of diet.

Every single one of us has an individual constitution (body type), therefore each of us requires different nutritional needs. Those needs are based on many different factors, and just like you those factors are constantly evolving and changing. The good thing is our bodies are always giving us signals and symptoms to guide us toward what to eat. Optimal health comes by having the wisdom to actually listen to those signals.

Your power resides in becoming aware of the connection between the foods you eat and the outcome it has on *your* body. Don't compare yourself to what others are eating or not eating. *One person's cure can be another person's poison.* Listen to *your* body. This means that even though something may be considered a "healthy food," it may not be right for you.

Starting now, I want you to check in with yourself after every meal and see how you feel. Begin to eat more of what feels good to you and less of what doesn't.

The food you eat can either be the safest and most powerful form of medicine, or the slowest form of poison. It is your job to find out what those foods are. Most medical doctors are not trained in nutrition, so they are left to prescribe you pharmaceuticals to cover up your problems. Not taking into consideration that most diseases and ailments can be cured by our own lifestyle choices.

The sicker you are or the greater change you desire, the stricter your diet needs to be.

Below are some modalities that I like to consider when looking at my diet. I do not live by just one rule or way. I like to find the common threads among many modalities and then report back to my body and see how it responds.

See if there are any common threads for you and begin to look at the connections between how you nourish your body and its effect on your overall health and well-being.

THE BLOOD TYPE DIET

The blood type diet is a revolutionary personalized diet system based on your blood type (a genetic fingerprint) that can help you to reach your ideal weight and slow down the aging process. Knowing your blood type is an important tool in understanding how your body responds to different foods, stress, and your susceptibility to certain diseases. It is a key genetic factor that influences your health and well-being. I have personally seen many people suffering from digestive disorders, headaches, and other ailments who have a full recovery once their diet was in line with their specific genetic fingerprint.

If you don't know your blood type, then you can easily get a blood test done from your doctor. You might find that you have naturally gravitated toward the foods specific for your blood type. I also highly recommend Dr. Peter D'Adamo's book *Eat Right 4 Your Type*.

The following is based on D'Adamo's system:

Type O: Meat-eater
Type Os do best with intense physical exercise. Their immune system is "environmentally intolerant" to foods such as grains and potatoes, which can cause inflammation. They have an overactive immune system, giving them the highest rate of cancer among all four blood types.

Type A: Vegetarian
Type As have a sensitive digestive tract but a tolerant immune system. They do best with centering exercises, such as yoga and tai chi, and are predisposed to diabetes, heart disease, and cancer.

Type B: Dairy-eater
Type Bs have the most flexible dietary choices. They do best with moderate exercise that requires mental balance, such as cycling or hiking. They have the strongest immune system and tend to resist most chronic degenerative diseases.

Type AB: Lean protein, organic vegetables, and grains
Type ABs have a sensitive digestive tract and immune system. This type is the most recent blood type in terms of evolution, and do it does the best with a combination of Type A and B suggestions.

Each blood type has a list of foods to avoid, foods that are beneficial, and foods that are moderate. I encourage you to dive deeper into seeing what foods benefit you most for your blood type and see if your body agrees.

AYURVEDA
Ayurveda is an ancient Indian modality that is based on three different types of bodily constitutions called doshas. Doshas are the energies that make up every individual.

They are composed from the five elements: ether, earth, water, fire, and air. Each dosha has certain physical features, personalities, sensitivities, and needs. Each person has all three doshas, but usually one is predominant and that is the one most susceptible to imbalances. The goal is to create a balanced diet and lifestyle that supports your unique nature.

The three doshas are:

Vata: Air + Ether (think wind)

- Governs all bodily movement.

- Tends to be thin and cold intolerant as well as having a light frame and a very active mind.

- Vata foods are grounding, warming, building, nourishing, and moist.

- When vata doshas are in balance, there is joy, creativity and vitality. When they are out of balance, there can be worry, stress, and fear.

Pitta: Fire + Water (think steam)

- Governs the transformation of food and ideas.

- Medium physique, strong build, hot in nature and tend to have a very intelligent and focused mind.

- Pitta foods are grounding, sustaining, cooling, calming and dry.

- Physical problems include bodily disorders such as constipation, as well as dry skin and hair.

- When pitta doshas are in balance, they are confident, intelligent, and focused. When they are out of balance, they can become irritated, aggressive, and pushy.

- Physical problems include inflammation of the skin—rashes, acne, boils, and skin cancer—along with insomnia, heartburn, and ulcers.

Kapha: Water + Earth (think mud)

- Governs the digestion of food and ideas.

- Soft, full features, sturdy, moist/oily, with a tendency to be very calm, slow, patient, and easygoing.

- Kapha foods are light, dry, well-spiced, warm, energizing, and easy to digest.

- When kapha doshas are in balance, they are very loving and affectionate. When they are out of balance, they can become possessive, insecure, and envious.

- Physical problems include respiratory issues, such as asthma, allergies, and sinus colds.

Opposites cure: We know that moving air fuels fire and that earth or water thrown on the fire will subdue it. Based on this profound yet basic principle, you can subdue or bring back in balance an aggravated dosha.

EAT LIKE YOUR ANCESTORS DID

Another factor to implement when deciding what foods are best for you is to find out what your ancestry is and what foods are native to that area of the world. For instance, if you have an Eastern European heritage, apples and berries would be appropriate, or if your ancestors were from the Pacific Islands, then pineapple, mango and sweet foods may be more suitable. If a person of Irish descent was living in a cold climate, regularly eating a lot of tropical fruit, it would create an imbalance in the body. Tropical fruit would be too expansive for someone of Irish decent, living in a climate where tropical fruit doesn't naturally grow. However, if that same person went on an island vacation, then it would be okay to eat tropical fruit. Your body adjusts best to a new environment when it eats foods from that environment.

Mother Nature has perfectly given us what we need for each climate and season. Try to eat with the season since that is when foods will be the freshest and contain nutrients that your body needs during that particular time of year. Just as locally grown foods are best assimilated into your body because they are grown in your own environment. Foods that you have grown yourself are the most beneficial for you as you put your own energy into the harvest of that food and that energy comes back to you tenfold, making the food the most nutritional for you and your loved ones.

YOU ARE WHAT YOU EAT

Every thirty-five days, your skin regenerates itself. Your liver, every six weeks. Your stomach, every five days. Your bones are constantly regenerating but the complete process takes ten years. Your body makes new cells from the food you eat. What you eat literally becomes you. You have a choice in what you're made of.

Every single food cultivates different energies into our bodies, some good and some bad. Depending on our constitution, time of year, origin of food, and health we can either be positively or negatively affected by our food choices. It is even believed that some people can be affected by the pain and suffering that animals have gone through to be slaughtered when consuming animal products.

Have you ever noticed how most vegetarians and health conscious eaters often have a calm, soft, kind spirit and those who have poor diet and lifestyle habits can become anxious, hard, or angry?

On the flip side, sometimes vegetarians can become too airy, leaving them lofty and not grounded. Balancing a clean diet with grounding practices, such as earthing, yoga, meditation, or a heavy crystal or rock in the pocket, is essential. Otherwise one can turn to sugar, smoking, or alcohol in a desire to attain the balance of such a clean diet. Too much outside stimulation can cause this same issue. That is one of the reasons it is recommended to refrain from watching television or being on your phone while eating or in a severe healing crisis.

The root of dis-ease and disruptions in the mind is an imbalance in the body. Our bodies are constantly seeking this perfect balance. A balance that is forever changing, so we must become adaptable, mindful, and open.

For instance, crunchy foods like chips, crackers, and cookies can make your body hard and acidic, which can turn your personality toward one who would be irrational and explosive. Softer foods like brown rice, sea vegetables, and soups help keep your body subtle and your spirit light.

Since our bodies cultivate the characteristics of each food we introduce to it, eat more of what you desire to cultivate and less of what you don't. Everything you put into your body matters. Once you start choosing more positive foods, the positive effects will start to appear.

Here is a breakdown of some common and maybe not so common foods and their reaction in the body.

POSITIVE

<u>Attraction, wisdom, consideration, and understanding:</u>
Millet, round vegetables, and natural sweets.

<u>Patience, endurance, adventure, and creativity:</u>
Leafy vegetables, miso soup, pickles, fermented foods, barley, and wheat.

<u>Confidence, courage, and inspiration:</u>
Buckwheat, adzuki beans, seaweed, sea salt, miso, and naturally salty foods.

<u>Gentleness, cooperation, quietness, intuition, humor, and joy:</u>
Big leafy vegetables, burdock, wakame, kombu, corn, and naturally bitter foods.

<u>Happiness, security, and integrity:</u>
Rice, broccoli, lotus root, cauliflower, daikon, ginger, and scallion.

NEGATIVE

<u>Irritable, critical, worrisome, jealous, and envious:</u>
Meat, eggs, butter, saturated and trans fat, cheese, milk, oil, sugar, white rice, and alcohol.

<u>Temperamental, angry, violent, cruel, stubborn, and intolerant:</u>
Meat, eggs, poultry, dairy, white flour, sugar, and alcohol.

<u>Fearful, defensive, lacking self-esteem, distant, cold, and desperate:</u>
Saturated and trans fat, oil, poultry, sugar, white flour, too much liquid, juices, cold foods, refined salt, refined oils, and drugs.

<u>Agitated, separate, hysterical, and talkative:</u>
Saturated and trans fats, oil, sugar, fruit and fruit juice, tropical foods, chemicals, coffee, and refined foods.

<u>Sad, depressed, indecisive, too analytical, confused, and weak:</u>
Meat, eggs, poultry, sugar, dairy, oil, white flour, spices, drugs, and tobacco.

The doctor of the future will give no medicine, but will interest his patients in the care of the human frame, in diet, and in the cause and prevention of disease.

—**THOMAS EDISON**

REFLECT

What is your blood type? List some foods that are most beneficial for your blood type.

_____

_____

_____

What type of foods are you going to eat more of based on your predominant dosha?

_____

_____

_____

What foods are native to your heritage?

_____

_____

_____

What foods are you going to eat more and less of based on the positive and negative characteristics of food?

_____

_____

_____

Eat 80/20

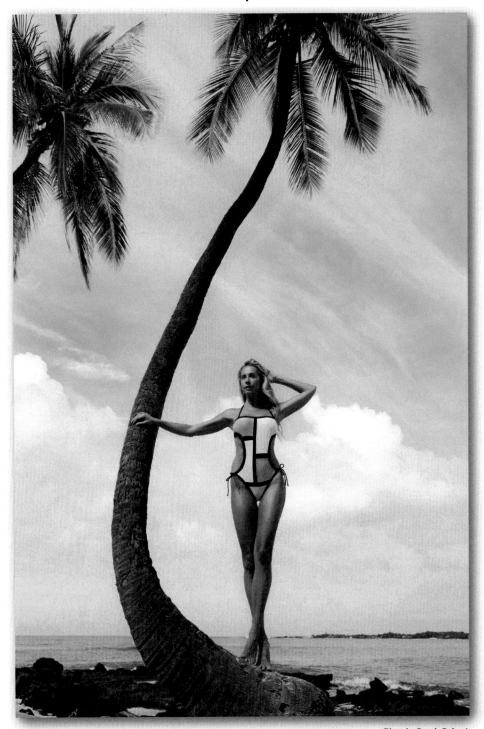

Photo by Sarah Orbanic

Life ought to be lived in balance. If you restrict your diet too much, then it can become too hard to maintain, causing your quality of life to be negatively affected. If you are too gluttonous, then your health will ultimately suffer and you will not perform at your optimal ability.

An easy way to describe "clean eating" is to ask you to imagine what you would eat prior to the dawn of the grocery store. Then, go into your grocery store, and notice that the perimeter of the store is where you will find the cleanest foods: fruits and vegetables, fresh grains, meat, and dairy. Most of the inner aisles are stocked with highly processed food items. Try to stick to the perimeter and choose brands that are fresh, local, organic, wild, free-range, antibiotic- and hormone-free, non-GMO, and without added preservatives or additives.

I have a Golden rule: only clean food is allowed at home. The energy of food in your house does matter. Not only will you be less tempted if it's not available to you, but the energy in your kitchen will ooze health and in turn keep you on your path. Splurge when you go out to dinner, the movies, or other people's homes, but do not allow junk food in the house. Junk food includes foods with artificial food coloring and flavor additives. Look for labels that state "artificial color added" or "made with artificial flavor" and steer clear.

Most European countries have banned these additives due to their potential to mutate healthy DNA. These artificial additives can also cause tumors of the nervous system. Food dyes derived from plants are the safe alternative.

The sicker you are, the cleaner your diet needs to be.

HOW TO EAT CLEAN:

- Eat *whole foods* that are natural and have not been tampered with in any way.

- Cook at home, from scratch, and avoid prepackaged goods that have been processed.

- Have each meal consist of a variety of fresh vegetables to ensure a variety of nutrients, ideally eating at least half of them raw.

- Eat adequate protein to maintain your strength: plant proteins, legumes, yogurt, wild fish, and/or free-range meats.

- Consume healthy grains that are high in fiber, such as brown rice, quinoa, or steel cut oats. I like to make brown rice every three to four days in order to have it on hand when craving more fullness. Brown rice will stabilize your blood sugar and be "glue" for your intestinal tract, helping to gather and eliminate toxins and waste.

- Enjoy seasonal fruits instead of refined sugar, but do keep fruit to a minimum as it is high in sugar content.

- Prepare healthy daily snacks with almonds and Brazil nuts, two of the most alkalizing nuts that exist.

- Make vegetable juices or broths in between meals, in place of a meal, or when your body feels like it, and rotate ingredients to ensure a well-rounded variety of nutritional benefits.

- Hydrate! The majority of our body is made up of water, so you need to replenish your body with adequate amounts of it. Drink six to eight glasses of clean, pure-quality water per day to help flush out harmful toxins and detoxify your system. Add lemon for an extra alkalizing effect to help balance your pH level (the measure of acidity and alkalinity in your body.)

MACROBIOTIC DIETARY GUIDELINES FOR TEMPERATE REGIONS:
Daily Regular Intake
40–50 percent whole grains
25–35 percent variety of vegetables
5–10 percent beans and sea vegetables
5–10 percent soups (various)

Weekly (a few to several times a week)
Fish and seafood (optional)
Local fruit, seeds, and nuts
Natural oils, seasonings, condiments, and sweets
Nonaromatic and nonstimulant beverages and occasional aromatic and stimulant beverages

Monthly (optional, infrequent, or transitional)
Meat
Eggs and poultry
Dairy

ACID/ALKALINE BALANCE

When the body is too acidic, disease thrives. When the body is alkaline, disease cannot live. The total pH (power of hydrogen) scale ranges from 1.0 to 14.0, with 7.0 being the perfect balance. Anything below 7.0 is considered to be acidic and anything above 7.0 is alkaline. Being too acidic causes your body to pull nutrients from other areas, like your bones, which can create inflammation, lactic acid, bone spurs, gout, and general ill health. When you are slightly alkaline and bring your body back into balance, disease cannot live. Cancer cannot live in the presence of oxygen. In this way, you can starve disease or feed it.

It takes an estimated ninety days for your body to go from acid to alkaline.

<u>ALKALINE</u>: 70-80 PERCENT OF YOUR DIET

Lemon, dark leafy greens, almonds, brazil nuts, lentils, lima beans, soy, millet, quinoa, buckwheat, spelt, seeds.

All vegetables are alkaline but there is a group of vegetables called nightshade vegetables that can cause inflammation in the body. These vegetables are tomatoes, eggplants, potatoes, bell and hot peppers (capsicum). People who have inflammation, such as arthritis, should steer clear from nightshade vegetables. This doesn't mean forever, but your body will tell you if you have a deterrent to it. For example, if you have to take antacids after eating red peppers, then that is your body telling you to stop eating them. If you suffer from arthritis and notice more inflammation in your joints after eating nightshade vegetables, then you need to decide what you love more…the nightshade vegetables (and resulting arthritis) or your being arthritis-free?

<u>ACID</u>: 20-30 PERCENT OF YOUR DIET

Sugar, wheat, aged cheese, caffeine, all other nuts, alcohol, tobacco, grains, legumes.

ALKALINE FOODS TO EAT MORE OFTEN:

Top three: celery, lemon, and cucumbers

Root vegetables: radishes, carrots, beets, turnips, and rutabagas

Cruciferous vegetables: cabbage, cauliflower, and broccoli

Leafy Greens: kale, spinach, Swiss chard, and turnip greens

Other: wheatgrass, cayenne peppers (capsicum), avocado, almonds, sprouts, chai seeds, watermelon, agar-agar, seaweed, garlic, and raw coconuts

Top anti-inflammatory foods: ginger, pineapple, papaya, bok choy, turmeric, aloe, shiitake mushrooms, leafy greens, garlic, fermented vegetables, and tea (matcha green tea)

If you eat clean 80 percent of the time, then you can afford to occasionally enjoy a cocktail or treat of your choice 20 percent of the time.

I believe moderation is the difference between healthy benefits and poison.

FOR THOSE WHO ENJOY WINE:
Research shows that one glass of wine a night can prolong life, diminish the risk of heart disease, and help you relax. I feel as if one glass of wine per night is a little excessive for me, so I like to drink herbal teas during the week to relax. I save drinking wine for nights that I go out on the town.

Doctors say no more than one glass of wine per day for women of all ages and for men over sixty-five, and no more than two glasses per day for men sixty-five and younger.

FOR THOSE WHO ENJOY CAFFEINE:
Personally, I love coffee. Most mornings it is my motivation to get up! Organic coffee, especially whole-bean black coffee and dark-roasted coffee, actually have many health benefits. Coffee contains compounds that have antioxidant and anti-inflammatory effects that have been shown to inhibit cancer cell growth. Coffee can also lower your risk for type 2 diabetes, stroke, Parkinson's disease, Alzheimer's disease, heart disease, and certain chronic diseases, all while giving your metabolism a boost and increasing your longevity. However, this does not include conventional coffees loaded with artificial sugars and creamers, and we must not overdo it, one to two cups at the most per day.

Chew Your Food Thoroughly

This may seem impossible at first, but one of the simplest ways to help your body's digestive system work properly is to chew your food until it is thoroughly liquefied.

No matter what you are eating, chewing thoroughly will slow down how fast you eat and give your body the time and ability to assimilate all the nutrients. Chewing also stimulates your brain and creates enzymes that break down your food for proper digestion.

Eating quickly puts your body into a stressed state and misses what scientists call "cephalic phase digestive response" (CPDR), an important digestive response that enables you to pleasurably taste your food. In order to taste your food, you need to slow down and consciously chew it.

HOW TO EAT MINDFULLY:

- Always eat sitting down. If you don't have time to sit down and eat, then wait until you do.

- Avoid your television, computer, smartphone, or any other electronic devices during meal times.

- Focus on what you are eating and whom you are eating with. Have gratitude for each bite and the food will be even more nutritious and digestible.

- Refrain from drinking too much liquid while you eat. Instead, sip lukewarm water if needed. The more you chew, the less you will need liquid while you eat and you will allow your body to assimilate the nutrients from your food properly.

- A proper meal, which ideally would fit comfortably in two cupped hands, should take thirty minutes to one hour to eat. I know what you are thinking, who has time to eat like that? My answer is, you do! You will create that time for yourself because your health depends on it and it will encourage proper meal times with loved ones.

Did you know that it takes your brain about twenty minutes after you start eating to even realize your stomach is full?

All it takes is overeating one meal a day to overburden your digestive system and affect the function of your colon. Adequately chewing your food gives your body time to realize it is full, thus avoiding this problem.

As my mother always said, "You don't have teeth in your stomach."

Intermittent Fasting

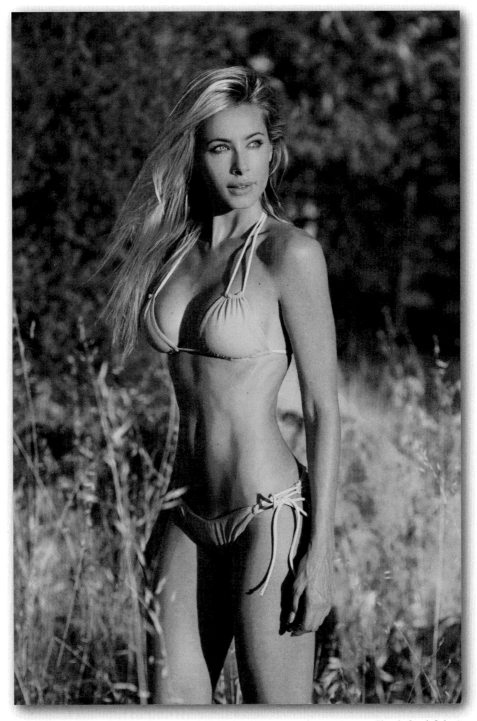

Photo by Sarah Orbanic

Looking back at how our ancestors ate, before obesity was an epidemic, people would go for long periods of time in between meals because they had to hunt and gather their food and did not have access to food 24/7, as we do now. Intermittent fasting (timing your food) is similar in that you eat your food during a specific window of time.

Intermittent fasting allows your body to shift into fat burning mode, promoting human growth hormone production, which can slow down the aging process and decrease inflammation and free radical damage. It is one of the "secrets" to optimizing your weight, and I believe is the "token to the fountain of youth."

Unlike most diets, intermittent fasting has nothing to do with calorie restriction or specific food choices, but more to do with how often and when you eat. Success with intermittent fasting is accomplished through daily behavioral changes.

HOW TO FAST MINDFULLY:
First, let go of the belief that you need three solid meals plus snacks. Unless you are training for a strong-man competition or another athletic endeavor where you desire to bulk up tremendously, there is no need for this much food. When you graze all day, you never give your body a chance to replenish itself, and contrary to popular belief, over time your body will forget how to burn fat as fuel, causing your metabolism to slow down and get lazy.

Once you get over the idea that you need to eat all the time, fasting is easy to implement and very effective.

THERE ARE SEVERAL DIFFERENT OPTIONS THAT YOU CAN TRY:

- **Eight-hour fasting**: Every day eat during an eight-hour window and fast the other remaining hours, which gives your body the time it needs to clean out all the garbage and regenerate. For example, only eat between the hours of 9:00 a.m. and 5:00 p.m., and after 5:00 p.m. sip herbal teas, warm water, or other healthy liquid options to keep you hydrated.

- **Six-hour fasting:** If eight-hour fasting feels good, shorten the window of time to eat to six hours per day. It should be a natural evolution, not something that is pushed, so notice how your body feels and reacts.

- **Skipping one meal:** Skip breakfast and have your first meal at noon and your second meal at 8:00 p.m. so that you are eating a total of two meals per day. If breakfast is your favorite meal, then just have it at lunchtime. Or shift the times and skip dinner. Refrain from eating two hours before vigorous exercise and have your last meal at least two hours before bed.

- **Alternating days**: Alternate between a day of intermittent fasting and a day of eating as you wish.

- **One day a week**: Choose one day a week that is ideal for you to fast and enjoy your regular eating schedule the other six days.

- **Nightly fasting**: Nightly fasting is just extending the natural fasted state that the body experiences while sleeping by refraining from eating two to five hours prior to bed.

It is not uncommon to have emotions arise when you first start fasting. Time and space open up when you are not busy eating all day, and it spiritually allows you the time to re-explore yourself.

After some time, your body will self-regulate and intuitively desire this fasting practice.

As I have gotten older, my body has naturally gravitated to this practice and I feel my strongest and best when I am diligent with it, especially with having rheumatoid arthritis. After some time of this fasting practice, our insulin levels normalize and insulin levels play a huge factor in fighting chronic diseases like rheumatoid arthritis and even cancer.

The practice of fasting requires discipline and patience. It frees you from your dependencies and allows your body, mind, and spirit to become clear.

It is about resetting your metabolism and it may take some time for your body to adapt, so be kind and patient with yourself.

Intermittent fasting is appropriate for most people, but if you are hypoglycemic or diabetic then you should be extra cautious before implementing this practice. Always talk to your doctor before starting any new diet or exercise. As for pregnant women, breastfeeding mothers, children under twenty years of age, people who are underweight, and those who have or have had an eating disorder, fasting is not for you.

Also, intermittent fasting does not include forgoing of proper hydration. In fact, it is ideal that you drink more, pure, clean water and other healthy liquids when fasting.

TIPS TO ACHIEVING A SUCCESSFUL FAST:

1. Stay hydrated

2. Choose the best days and times for your schedule.

3. Stay active but don't overdo it.

4. Spend time outside getting fresh air and sun.

5. Get plenty of rest.

6. Make sure your meals consist of healthy foods.

7. Reward yourself.

This practice should make you feel good. If you are feeling weak instead of strong then step back and moderate your fast.

Plant-based Diet

Nothing will benefit human health and increase the chances for survival of life on Earth as much as the evolution to a vegetarian diet.

—*ALBERT EINSTEIN*

I believe that there is nothing better that you could do for your health than to switch to a plant-based diet.

I'm not saying you need to stop eating all animal products, *although that is ideal*, but I am suggesting that you start eating plant-based meals several times a week. The meat industry is a "supply and demand" market, so eating fewer animal products causes fewer animals to be killed, and a vegetarian diet requires only one third of the land needed to support a meat and dairy diet. I believe a certain number of animals are saved every time you choose to forgo eating meat. In fact, it is estimated that, on average, a person can save eight cows in one month, a hundred in a year, and three hundred in three years by choosing to forgo beef.

We are conditioned to think that meat is good for us and that we need the protein to survive. It's just not true, and meanwhile we are poisoning ourselves and increasing our risk of diseases like cancer and heart disease, which is the number one killer of men and women. So much of what we think about food and nutrition is told to us by people who are benefiting most by the misinformation.

Every day, billions of animals are being slaughtered in unbelievable conditions. I guarantee you that if you saw where half of the meat and animal products you ate came from, you would stop eating it altogether. The problem is we choose to turn a blind eye and think that it's survival and just a part of the circle of life. Unless you are in such a remote area where there is no vegetation and hunting your food is your only option, eating meat is a choice. It is not a necessity.

Humans are the most successful species on the planet and that is because we are survivors. We have survived because of food made by Mother Nature. Yes, we were hunters *and* gatherers, but we survived for *most* of that time as gatherers. Before chronic disease, heart disease, cancers, and inflammatory arthritic disease, only a certain class of people could afford animal meats. Now they are so readily available and in excess. Instead of having the main meal be plant-based, it is animal-based with a couple of side vegetables. The foods that matter are plants, not meat. We do it backward. Eat your veggies first and most often! The human requirement for protein each day can be easily filled with plants. We do not need as much protein as we have been told.

Despite the myth that you need animal protein to survive, it is almost impossible to have a protein deficiency when you eat the proper caloric and variety of plant-based foods. A well-thought-out plant-based diet is rich in protein, iron, calcium, and other essential vitamins and minerals. Sources of these nutrients tend to be low in saturated fat, high in fiber, and packed with antioxidants, mitigating some of the modern world's biggest health issues like obesity, heart disease, diabetes, and cancer, which animal protein actually fuel.

What about calcium? A big kale salad provides more calcium that one glass of milk, and three ounces of chia seeds meets more than half of the suggested requirement. Milk is great…if you're a baby calf! We are the only mammals that drink another mammal's milk. Think about it. Cow milk is not designed for human consumption. It is made to breastfeed a baby calf so that the calf can become a cow. Elimination of all dairy products can clear up a plethora of health issues after just one month. Try a healthy alternative to cow milk, such as almond, hemp, or coconut milk.

Foregoing red meat is a great start, too, but don't fool yourself into thinking you can then eat more chicken, turkey, and fish. They are just as bad and sometimes can be worse. Most of the fish we eat are high on the food chain and filled with mercury and other pollutants.

IF YOU CAN'T DO IT FOR YOURSELF, DO IT FOR THE PLANET.
In addition to your own health being impacted positively, choosing to eat less meat also has a huge impact on the environment. So if you are not able to do it for yourself, do it for the planet! Avoiding all animal products is one of the most effective things you can do to lower your carbon footprint.

According to a 2006 report published by the United Nations Food and Agriculture Organization, the livestock sector generates more greenhouse gas emissions than transportation. It is also a major source of land and water degradation, causing it to be one of the most significant contributors to today's most serious environmental problems.

When it comes to water shortages and droughts, taking quick showers and watering your lawn less is of minimal help in comparison to having a veggie burger instead of a beef burger.

It takes 880 to 1,000 gallons of water to produce just one gallon of milk! And it takes 2,500 gallons of water to produce one pound of beef! Do you know why? Because you need water to raise, graze, feed, irrigate, and process the beef.

The more we demand to have these vegetarian and vegan options in our markets, the more available and cost effective they will become. This movement has grown leaps and bounds since I declared being a vegetarian at eleven years old, and it is because consumers as a whole have demanded it. The possibility for change starts with one person…you.

Livestock (farmed animals) are key players in the emergence of antibiotic resistance. If you do eat meat, choose antibiotic-free, free-range, organic, and hormone-free, or better yet hunt it yourself. People eat meat and think they will become as "strong as an ox," forgetting that the oxen eat grass.

SO WHAT *DO* WE EAT?
Don't get stressed or overwhelmed thinking that you will have to give up all your favorite foods all at once. There will be a transition period and at first you will miss some of your animal proteins, but with time your body *will* adjust, and in your renewed health, you will start to crave plant-based foods.

- Start with the plant-based foods you already eat and begin to create meals based on those.

- Eat seasonally. Everything in nature is designed perfectly for us. The foods that grow during each season carry the nutrients we need most during that time.

- Overall the best plant-based diet for humans comes from four foods groups: fruit, vegetables, whole grains, and legumes. Low in fat and high in fiber, your overall diet should ideally be 90–95 percent plant-based.

- Add more legumes to your diet by trying meat alternatives like seitan, tempeh, and organic soy, available at most grocery stores now. When buying soy products, be sure they are organic, as soy is one of the most genetically modified foods in the United States.

Notice how you feel after a vegan meal versus a nonvegan meal. I promise you will feel nourished, lighter, more energetic, and more clearheaded. Along with the health benefits you will reap, you will also be contributing to the preservation of our environment.

When non-vegetarians say that "human problems come first," I cannot help wondering what exactly it is that they are doing for human beings that compels them to continue to support the wasteful, ruthless exploitation of farm animals.

—**PETER SINGER, ANIMAL LIBERATION**

Gluten-free Diet

I know, I know, it seems as if everybody is on a gluten-free diet these days, but there is good reason. In my opinion, gluten is *no bueno* for anybody. It is known to create inflammation in the body and fuel heart disease, Alzheimer's disease, high cholesterol, and even cancer.

Gluten is a protein found in certain grains, such as wheat, spelt, barley, and rye. *Why are so many people gluten intolerant?* Health professionals say one of the reasons may be that in the last hundred years, we have reversed what we are naturally supposed to eat, like babies eating carbohydrates and grown adults drinking milk. If babies are given starch (rice cereals, oatmeal, crackers) prior to having their molars, for example, it can throw off the balance of bacteria in their gut and lead to all kinds of complications as they age, including food allergies. Molars produce p*tyalin*, an enzyme in the saliva that breaks down carbohydrates. Without molars, undigested grains are left to wreak havoc on a babies' intestinal lining.

Another reason many people are gluten intolerant is that we eat more grain with gluten than ever before. Gluten binds the grains so that they won't break and so that they look pretty on the grocery store shelf.

Even if you feel as if you are not directly affected with an autoimmune disease, like celiac or Hashimoto's, where the effect of gluten can be instantaneous, I suggest limiting and finding better, healthier alternatives to gluten.

Gluten-free options: Amaranth seed, buckwheat, flaxseed, millet, rice (brown preferred), sorghum, and quinoa.

Many gluten-free products contain corn, which is one of the most genetically modified foods in the United States, so read packages and look for non-GMO, organic corn options.

If you do notice stomach problems when eating gluten, it may be that you are eating it at the same time as protein, which, for some people, creates inadequate digestion and assimilation. Eating these foods separately is an option to try.

Try being gluten-free for a week and I promise you that you will feel less bloated, less lethargic, more clearheaded, and more energetic, and your skin may even reap the rewards with a little glow.

Often what we love most is what causes us the most problems.

Superfoods

All foods are *not* created equal. There are certain foods that are loaded with an abundance of vitamins, trace minerals, and amino acids that our bodies need for optimal health. With the ability to trim your waistline, restore your energy levels, and make your skin glow, I suggest incorporating some of these foods into your daily diet. Keeping in mind that variety and moderation are key.

HERE ARE MY FAVORITE SUPERFOODS:

1. **Bee Pollen**:

   - Contains an abundance of B vitamins, as well as vitamins C, A, and E, folic acid, protein, and amino acids.

   - Acts as a transporter to carry nutrients into the bloodstream and is used as an effective muscle recovery and endurance booster for many Olympic athletes.

   - The average recommended daily dose is one to two tablespoons per day.

2. **Spirulina:**

   - Spirulina is a blue-green algae that provides all eight essential amino acids vitamins A, E, F, and B-complex, and chlorophyll.

   - With 60 percent protein, spirulina is the highest of any plant-based food (beef contains only 22 percent)!

   - Also acts as an internal deodorant for your body and breath.

   - There are some contradictions for people who have phenylketonuria or an autoimmune disorder so always speak with your doctor before taking spirulina or any supplement. Easily added to any green drink or smoothie, or taken alone.

3. **Sea Vegetables**:

   - Traditionally used in oriental medicine, seaweed has all fifty-six minerals and trace minerals necessary for optimal body function.

- Seaweed is antiviral and antibacterial, strengthens the immune system, reduces cholesterol, lowers blood pressure, and improves metabolism and digestion.

- Also contains calcium phosphate, which helps in the prevention of osteoporosis, and calcium, along with natural iodine, which can lower the risk of cancer and thyroid dysfunction.

The future of nutrition is found in the ocean.

—*Jacques-Yves Cousteau*

4. **Coconut:**

- This "creation from the heavens" tastes amazing and contains important electrolytes and trace minerals, along with proteins, fiber, fatty acids, and other vitamins to replenish and hydrate, internally and externally.

- Has been used for many purposes and is revered as one of the greatest superfoods of all time.

- Coconut water is almost identical to that of human blood plasma, which is about 55 percent of our blood composition. A natural energy source, coconut water is high in MCT (medium-chain triglycerides), a key component to any longevity and optimal health plan.

- Capable of jump-starting your metabolism and regulating your hormones, coconuts and coconut oil can also help you attain your optimal weight.

- Coconut oil is a great oil to cook with as it is a high-heat oil. You can also add it to your smoothies, coffee, or tea.

5. **Aloe Vera:**

- The long history of aloe vera expands from Alexander the Great to Egyptian queens like Nefertiti and Cleopatra. This sturdy plant has been used for centuries in many cultures for longevity, beauty regimens, and religious ceremonies.

- Can be used internally and externally for a variety of ailments. It is immune boosting, anti-inflammatory, antifungal, and antiviral.

- Capable of DNA repair, this soothing plant supports the replication of cells responsible for our connective tissues, making it an optimal superfood to add to your diet.

- Rich in chemical compounds that speed up healing by arresting pain and inflammation, it stimulates the immune system and encourages cellular repair.

- Aloe has a laxative effect that can help the body to properly eliminate. I like to drink one to two ounces before bed as it promotes elimination by the morning.

6. **Fermented Vegetables**:

- Eat them and eat them often. As I talk about in the probiotics chapter, most of us have damaged gut flora and lack healthy beneficial bacteria. Fermented vegetables are one of the most beneficial ways to provide your body with healthy bacteria.

7. **Chai Seeds**:

- Aztec warriors used carbohydrate-rich chai seeds as an energy booster.

- High in fiber and loaded with essential key nutrients and essential amino acids, they are a complete form of protein. An ancient dietary staple that has withheld the test of time.

- Many athletes and health conscious people eat chia seeds because once placed in water, the seeds increase in weight and size without any added calories, tricking your body into thinking it is full for hours.

8. **Hemp seeds**:

- Produced by the hemp plant, *Cannabis sativa L.*, which is in the same family as marijuana, minus the THC (*tetrahydrocannabinol*) factor that gets you high.

- Hemp seeds are high in nutritional value. They contain twenty different amino acids and all nine of the essential amino acids that can't naturally be produced by the body.

- Hemp seeds also contain a balanced ratio of omegas and are another bioavailable complete protein.

Antioxidants are antiaging, youth-activating, disease-preventing, free radical fighters.

HERE ARE MY TOP THREE:

9. **Turmeric**:

- Turmeric's yellow pigments are known as curcuminoids, one of which is curcumin, the herb's most active ingredient.

- Has long been used in Ayurvedic medicine for a variety of ailments, from digestive disorders to infections of the skin, such as athlete's foot, eczema, and psoriasis.

- Is a natural anti-inflammatory and effective against both acute and chronic pain. Herbal practitioners also often recommend it for rheumatoid arthritis and osteoarthritis. (In experiments with rats, turmeric appeared to block inflammatory pathways associated with rheumatoid arthritis. Scientific studies also reveal that turmeric may rival hydrocortisone for reducing pain and stiffness associated with various forms of arthritis.)

- Turmeric has been shown to positively influence over seven hundred genes and is included in suggested treatment for certain types of cancers, prevention of cardiovascular disease, and reducing cholesterol.

- Add turmeric to teas, stews, and soups. Take it in supplement form or add it as an extra zesty seasoning to any meal.

10. **Green tea**:

- A potent antioxidant compound (EGCG) that is rich in flavonoids that has anticarcinogenic and anti-inflammatory properties.

- Studies suggest green tea may protect against cholesterol damage and may help to prevent blood clots and heart disease. It also has been shown to inhabit cancer growth.

- Green tea can also help regulate blood sugar as well as burn fat to aid in weight loss.

- Just one cup of green tea each day offers some "superpower" protection and can help you maintain your ideal weight!

11. **Resveratrol**:

- Naturally found in grapes, raspberries, mulberries, raw cacao, peanuts, and red wine (in abundance). (However, you would have to drink an excessive amount of red wine to get enough resveratrol to benefit you, and this excessive drinking would do more harm than good for your body. There is more resveratrol in red wine than white wine, but the benefit is from the grapes, so I recommend eating grapes or fresh grape juice to receive the benefits of resveratrol.)

- Resveratrol can help prevent heart disease, inhibits the formation and spread of cancerous tumors, and reduces the risk of Alzheimer's disease and depression.

- With chemical-detoxifying and anti-inflammatory properties, resveratrol combats free radicals in the body that make it a powerful force for life extension.

- There are also some studies that suggest this antioxidant might also protect you from diabetes and obesity.

Not all food is created equal. If you want to have "superpowers," you need to fuel your body with super antioxidant foods.

Probiotics

If I had to choose *just one* dietary supplement to take, that I have reaped the most benefit from, it would be probiotics. Of course, it is always best to try and get most of our nutrients from our food; however, taking a probiotic supplement can enrich your diet and help with chronic ailments.

Probiotics help create healthy gut flora in the stomach, and most people have damaged gut flora these days. This lack of healthy gut flora can be very damaging considering 80 percent of our immune system resides in our gut. Because of this fact, many health professionals believe that disease starts in the gut. The damaged gut flora is caused by overuse of antibiotics and poor food choices.

If you suffer from any digestive disorders, chronic illnesses, gas, belching, or bloating, then I would look into probiotics as an option. Probiotics can also play a significant role in alleviating mood disorders and help normalize your weight and reduce belly fat!

Lack of beneficial bacteria in the intestines can cause stomach issues like diarrhea or irregular bowel movements, bloating, the overgrowth of yeast, and even inflammation of the body, which can cause immune issues. Therefore, healthy flora in your intestines can help prevent and cure these issues.

Don't be fooled into just eating yogurt all the time either. Although yogurt has billions of healthy bacteria in it, it is often also loaded with added sugar. Be sure to check the sugar content on the label of the container before consuming.

If you get frequent urinary tract or vaginal infections, then staying on a regular probiotic can be extremely beneficial for you. You can even insert certain over-the-counter probiotics directly into your vagina for instant relief from a yeast infection. These probiotic products increase healthy bacteria to solve the problem, not cover it up.

Probiotics gently break up digestive waste by promoting regular elimination and are "magic" to the immune system and to any inflammation in the body, whether it be arthritis, eczema, lupus, multiple sclerosis, fibromyalgia, allergies, diabetes, chronic skin conditions, or degenerative diseases. All these diseases and conditions can be treated and, in some cases, healed from regular use of probiotics.

If disease does start in the gut, then as your digestive tract heals, symptoms will start to vanish within a couple of weeks.

Fermented foods, such as kefir (fermented milk), kombucha (fermented tea), kimchi (a Korean side dish of spicy fermented vegetables), and miso (fermented soybeans), are some of the best ways to provide your body with beneficial bacteria. Fermented foods also act as potent detoxifiers, as they draw out a wide range of toxins and heavy metals from the body.

Before grocery stores, many people would ferment vegetables and store them in glass jars for the winter. The fermented cabbage and other veggies helped keep their immune system strong during the cold winters, helping to prevent many illnesses associated with the colder months.

In the rare case that you do find yourself having to take antibiotics for a bacterial infection then it is recommended to take probiotics after the course of antibiotics to replace and rebalance the healthy bacteria that was destroyed from antibiotics.

The path to optimal health is paved with a good digestive tract.

Eat Fat

Yes, fat! Many people are afraid of fat and believe that consuming fat-free products is better for them.

Fact: If a food label says "fat-free," then the product is often loaded with hidden sugars and preservatives.

Now, I am not talking about eating saturated fats or trans fats found in many commercially packaged foods. I'm talking about the good fats: monounsaturated and polyunsaturated fats found in nuts, avocados, olive oil, flaxseed oil, sea vegetables, and cold-water fish.

These fats will actually increase your chances of weight loss and help you lose belly fat. In fact, one of the signs of essential fatty acid deficiency is the inability to lose fat! These fats are also responsible for keeping your hair shiny and your skin glowing.

Some of the healthiest populations in the world are known to consume the most healthy fats, including omega-3's, like in Japan and in the Mediterranean. Both regions consume a standard diet of fish, sea vegetables, whole grains, and other fresh produce. Their diets are believed to have about eight times the amount of omega-3s that you would find in a standard American diet. The lower ratio of omega-6s to omega-3s seems to be a key factor in reducing the risks of many chronic diseases that are becoming an epidemic in Western society.

Fats are essential for optimal health, hence the name *essential* fatty acids.

Omega-3 is an essential fatty acid that our body does not create, so we have to supplement it through our diet. The health benefits of omega-3s range from decreasing inflammation in joints to increasing cell proliferation (cell growth). Having about five grams of omega-3 oils per day in your diet has shown to help rheumatoid arthritis patients go into remission. They are also believed to help regulate your mood and hormone production.

On the contrary, we often consume too much omega-6, which comes from refined oils, extracted from grains and seeds like canola, sunflower, and grape-seed oil. Omega-6s create inflammation, arthritis, depression, and higher risk for heart disease, the opposite effect on our bodies from omega-3s.

It is best to lower your omega-6 intake and up the food sources that contain omega-3s into your diet.

TRY THESE SOURCES FOR OMEGA-3S:

Wild, cold-water fish: Fish is one the best sources for omega-3 fatty acids but there are plenty of vegan options available. In moderation, add small amounts to a meal for added nutrition and taste. Up to once a week to once a month, choose salmon, sardines, herring, black cod, anchovies, mackerel, blue fish, or lake trout. Wild fish has more omega-3s than farmed fish. I stay away from farmed fish because I believe farm-raised fish is more harmful than beneficial for one's health. The larger the fish, the more toxic the mercury content. Overfishing of certain fish has led to near extinction of some species, so eat only what is in abundance and dolphin/turtle safe.

Ghee: A clarified butter used in many Ayurveda recipes, ghee is composed almost entirely of fat, but it is considered a healthy alternative to butter. Ghee has numerous benefits, from improving your skin to increasing clarity of the mind to aiding in digestion to helping lose unwanted weight. I love ghee and often add a teaspoon of it to my coffee. Yes, coffee! Give it a try!

Coconuts and coconut oil: As I said before, I believe that coconuts are the cure-all for many things…internally and externally. The fat content in coconut oil has antiviral and antibacterial properties, and the fatty acids can stimulate your metabolism. This amazing creation from the heavens not only tastes great, but it also contains important electrolytes and trace minerals, along with proteins, fiber, fatty acids, and other vitamins to replenish and hydrate.

Fresh ground flaxseed and flaxseed oil: One of the richest sources of essential fatty acids, flaxseed has laxative effects, helps to sooth the digestive tract, and has anti-inflammatory properties. It is high in protein, fiber, calcium, iron, magnesium, and phosphorus, along with many other beneficial nutrients and essential amino acids. Add flaxseed oil to juices, salad dressing, and soups, or sprinkle the ground flaxseed on cereals or blend into smoothies. Flaxseed is a healthy thing to also add to your child's food without him or her noticing. Adequate omega-3 in a child's diet is proven to help with asthma, ADHD, and even depression. A teaspoon of ground flax has about 0.4 grams of omega-3 oil and about two grams of fiber. Hemp seeds also contain a balanced ratio of omegas.

Nuts and nut butter: An ounce of walnuts has 1.5 to 2 grams of omega-3 oils. Macadamia nuts and pecans have the largest amount of healthy fat, but all nuts make for a healthy snack. They contain valuable vitamins and minerals and are associated with a reduction in cancer and heart disease. Add walnuts to your oatmeal or eat raw almonds as a snack. Skip the conventional peanut butter, like Skippy's, which is high in trans-fat, and choose walnut, almond, macadamia, or cashew butters instead.

Cooking oil: When cooking with high heat, I would not use olive oil as it has a low smoke point, which means you could lose its health benefits and it may become harmful. The higher the smoke point, the better for you to cook with. I recommend coconut, avocado, or organic canola oils. (Most canola seeds are genetically modified in the United States so read your labels and be sure to buy GMO-free, organic canola oil.)

Avocados: Rich in essential nutrients and monounsaturated fat that turn into energy and enhances the body's ability to absorb other nutrients, avocados are linked to lowering the risk for diabetes and cardiovascular disease and improved weight management.

Often when you are craving carbohydrates it is a sign that you haven't had a sufficient amount of healthy fats in your diet.

Every Meal Is an Opportunity
to Be Healthier

HERE ARE SOME GUIDELINES TO USE TO BEGIN MOVING TOWARD
HEALTHIER EATING:

- Eat local, in season, and organic foods, which are healthy choices for you and the environment.

- Drink at least eight eight-ounce glasses of water per day. Ditch the bottled water and instead invest in a good home water filter. Purchase an aluminum, glass, stainless steel, or BPA-free plastic reusable bottle to refill daily.

- Focus on whole organic foods. When you do this, you don't have to ever count calories again and you will feel better than ever.

- Eat at least a third of your diet in the form of raw foods.

- Eat all the colors of the rainbow. Try not to eat the same things multiple days in a row. Variety is key.

- Rotate vegetables and fruit to receive the most nutrients from your diet. When your body does not get the sufficient nutrients it needs, it can pull from another source and the source could be toxic, as in radiation, lead, mercury. When your body is receiving and assimilating all the nutrients it needs, it is less likely to absorb harsh chemicals and toxins.

- Eat the colorful foods on your plate first, brown foods last. Eating your vegetables and proteins before carbohydrates can keep you fuller for a longer period of time.

- Have your biggest meal be your first meal and eat smaller meals as the day goes on.

- When eating animal protein, only eat organic, free-range or wild, antibiotic- and hormone-free options.

- Shop local farmer's markets for fresh produce. Your food *should* spoil in a couple of days; if it doesn't, chances are it isn't any good for you.

SWITCH IT OUT:

- Plant-based instead of animal-based

- Almond milk instead of cow milk

- Brown rice instead of white rice

- Homemade salad dressing with ingredients like olive oil, tahini, apple cider vinegar, lemon, and herbs instead of store bought salad dressings

- Whole wheat, spelt, millet, or amaranth instead of refined white flour

- Mustard instead of ketchup

- Miso soup instead of chicken soup

- Sea salt instead of processed table salt *(craving salt is a sign your body is lacking essential and trace minerals found in sea salt, not table salt.)*

JUST SAY NO:

- Ditch the soda, which includes diet soda! It could possibly be one of the worst things for you! Two or more cans a day increases your waistline by 500 percent!

- Absolutely no fast food. This stuff is not even food! It's dead! Eat live food. Remember, you are what you eat, so don't be fast, cheap, easy, or fake!

- Eliminate any processed additives and artificial preservatives, flavors, and colors.

- No artificial sweeteners or high fructose corn syrup, instead try stevia, honey, brown rice syrup, or raw sugar. Artificial sweeteners trick your body, making you crave more sugar.

- Fruit contains sugar, so treat it as such. It should be looked upon as a reward and best to eat the pure fruit itself (in order to also get its fiber) than a glass of fruit juice.

- No more than three cups of coffee a day max. Coffee can be great for your metabolism but drink too much and it will do the complete opposite. Ideally one to two cups are adequate.

- Ditch the ice. Drink room temperature water and teas.

- Avoid aluminum and Teflon pans. Instead use stainless steel, cast iron, or nabe pots (earthenware/clay).

- Ditch the microwave! There is no need to have one. I haven't had one for over fifteen years. Anything worth eating can be cooked on a natural gas stove or natural source.

GOING THE EXTRA MILE:

- Try to buy organic fruits and vegetables when possible, but if you cannot find them then soak your vegetables in a natural vegetable wash (or a couple drops of grape-seed extract added to water) to clean off any pesticides. Don't forgo eating fruits and vegetables because you can't find organic options. They will still be more nutritious than anything else you would replace them with. This is just one of the other magical things about fruits and vegetables, you can wash them, unlike packaged food or animal products.

- Make brown rice or quinoa every three to four days to have on hand to add to meals and when craving more fullness. It will stabilize your blood sugar and act like glue for your intestinal tract, helping to gather and eliminate waste from your body.

- Steaming should be your best friend. No frying in butter or oil. Steam rice, veggies, and even fish by wrapping it inside of a cabbage leaf! And you can reheat food in your steamer minus the radiation! (Again, ditch the microwave!)

- Flash cook vegetables to make them soft. Boil a little bit of water in a sauce pan and place the vegetables, broccoli for instance, in the boiling water for about thirty seconds or until bright green. Do not overcook them, as they will lose the nutritional values.

- You will see that all vegetables turn a brighter color when cooked perfectly, which is your cue that they are ready.

- Use herbs like cilantro and parsley for added flavor and aiding in removal of heavy metals from your body.

- Only take supplements that you know you are lacking or deficient in. Your body was designed to utilize nutrients from your diet, found in nature not a lab.

Internal Remedies

These are not your average smoothie recipes, which luckily seem to be readily available to everyone these days. I wanted to share with you recipes that you might not have ever seen before. These are recipes that became remedies and were a big part of my healing journey with rheumatoid arthritis and ones that I still use today. Many of these recipes are based on macrobiotic principles with some interesting and new ingredients, but they are easy to make and very effective. Old wisdom that has surpassed the test of time.

As with everything, listen to your body and strive for balance through moderation. The energy you put into your food matters. Make it positive! Recite positive affirmations while preparing these recipes and put love into everything you put into your body.

SWEET VEGGIE DRINK

This is a great drink for softening tightness in the body caused by poor food choices and heavy animal consumption. It also helps stabilize blood sugar levels and is especially beneficial for softening the pancreas and relaxing all the muscles of the body.

1. Choose four sweet vegetables, such as carrots, cabbage, onions, winter squash or *kabocha* (Japanese squash), depending on what is available. Finely chop all the vegetables and place into a big pot.

2. Add enough water to cover the vegetables and bring to a boil for two to three minutes. Reduce flame, cover, and simmer for twenty minutes.

3. Strain vegetables and set aside, for later use if desired.

4. Drink the broth hot or at room temperature.

5. Do not keep in the refrigerator for more than three or four days.

The ideal times to drink this is 3:00 p.m. and/or after a light dinner.

BLACK SOYBEAN TEA

This tea is great for warming the body, creating smooth bowel movements, and helping to shed excess fat from the body. Be sure to rinse your mouth after drinking, as the tea can stain your teeth.

1. Place one cup of black soybeans in a pot and add four cups of water.

2. Add a two-inch strip of *kombu* (seaweed) that has been soaked and finely chopped, then bring to a boil.

3. Cover and simmer for thirty to forty minutes.

4. Strain the beans and drink one cup of the dark, slightly sweet tea.

5. You may continue cooking beans until soft to use later for another meal.

6. Once cooled, place the remainder into the refrigerator and drink for the next four days.

7. Drink one cup per day maximum.

UME-SHO-KUZU DRINK

This drink is known to be highly alkaline-forming, therefore it is used for acidic conditions that cause headaches, indigestion, and even hangovers. Helps to restore energy and strengthen and promote good digestion. Also known to relieve migraines and muscular aches.

1. Dissolve one heaping teaspoon of powered *kuzu* (a Japanese mountain root vegetable) in two to three tablespoons of cold water.

2. Once it has dissolved, add one cup of cold water.

3. Add the pulp of one half to one whole *umeboshi* (a Japanese pickled and dried plum) that has been chopped and ground to paste.

4. Put all contents into a sauce pan and bring to a boil, stirring constantly to avoid lumping.

5. Once the liquid becomes translucent, reduce the flame to as low as possible.

6. Add several drops to one-half teaspoon of shoyu/soy sauce (gluten-free) and gently stir.

7. Simmer for two to three minutes.

8. Best to drink while it is hot.

SHIITAKE DRINK

Traditionally used to reduce fevers, dissolve animal fat, and to help relax a contracted or tight condition in the body. Dried shiitake mushrooms are preferred over fresh.

1. In a sauce pan, soak one dried shiitake mushroom into one cup of water for twenty to thirty minutes.

2. Once the shiitake is soft, chop it finely and return it to the water.

3. Bring to a boil.

4. Reduce the flame and simmer for ten to fifteen minutes.

5. Add a pinch of sea salt or a few drops of shoyu/soy sauce.

6. Best to drink while hot.

LOTUS ROOT TEA

This tea is good to relieve lung congestion, clear up sinus problems, and help to ease chronic coughing. This tea is most effective when used with fresh lotus root. However, if fresh is not available, you may use dried lotus root or lotus root powder.

With fresh lotus root:

1. Wash the lotus root and grate one-half cup.

2. Place the pulp into a piece of cheesecloth and squeeze out the juice into a sauce pan.

3. Add an equal amount of water to the lotus root juice.

4. Add a pinch of salt or a few drops of shoyu/soy sauce.

5. Bring to a boil and let simmer on a low flame for two to three minutes.

6. The tea will become thick and creamy and is best to drink while hot.

7. You may also add a few drops of grated ginger juice toward the end if you like.

With dried lotus root:

1. Place one-third ounce (about ten grams) of dried lotus root into one cup of water. Let it sit for a few minutes, until it gets soft.

2. Finely chop and mash in a *suribachi* (a Japanese mortar and pestle).

3. Return the lotus root to the soaking water and add a pinch of sea salt or a few drops of shoyu/soy sauce.

4. Bring to a boil and allow to gently simmer for approximately fifteen minutes.

5. Best to drink hot.

CARROT, CELERY, AND FLORENCE FENNEL/ANISE JUICE

Triple support for the heart, muscles, and skin as well as an electrolyte builder. Carrots are an excellent potassium booster, while celery is an excellent source of organic sodium. Fennel is filled with both potassium and sodium, along with sulphur. Great as an after exercise drink as it helps replenish electrolytes in the body. Drinking lots of carrot juice could give you an orange hue but many believe this is a sign that the liver is detoxifying itself through the pores. If this is the case, then you can always lessen the carrot juice and add more fennel. Don't worry, you will not stay orange forever and you may actually enjoy the golden hue to your skin tone.

1. Depending on your needs for more potassium (carrots) or more sodium (celery), base the ratio of carrot to celery on that and add a little fennel to taste.

2. If you do not know which you need more of, then use equal parts carrot/celery and add a little fennel.

3. Wash vegetables thoroughly and add desired amount into a Juicer or a Vitamix blender.

4. Drink four to eight ounces per day in between meals.

APPLE CIDER VINEGAR, TURMERIC, TANGERINE, OR LEMON JUICE WITH CHAI SEEDS

Upon waking up in the morning make one cup of this alkalizing ultimate cleanser. Known to fight inflammation, remove toxins, and help you to achieve your optimal weight.

1. Boil some water in a kettle or on the stove top.

2. Grate some turmeric (about the size of your thumb), wrap it in cheesecloth, and squeeze the turmeric juice into a clean coffee cup.

3. Put up to two tablespoons of apple cider vinegar into the cup with turmeric.

4. Add juice from a lemon or tangerine and a tablespoon of chai seeds.

5. Then add boiling water to fill the crest of the cup. If adding chai seeds, wait five minutes before drinking so that seeds have some time to plump up. Feel free to have another cup two hours prior to bed.

Raw, unfiltered, unpasteurized, organic apple cider vinegar is known for balancing the body's pH levels, clearing the skin, and even helping aid in weight loss.

The ritual of making a cup of tea is also very healing: The process of choosing a tea, preparing it, waiting for it to steep, and then holding the warm cup in your hands. Feeling the aromatic steam on your face as you deeply inhale. Everything about tea encourages mindfulness. It makes you pause and do something kind for yourself or your loved ones. It creates a moment of togetherness.

I always have a pot of tea on and I prefer loose leaf. I have a tea pot with a tea strainer inside of it, so it makes it easy to make a pot for the day. There are many teas to choose from and all with a unique purpose. The following are two of my favorites that don't get the recognition they deserve.

BANCHA TEA (*Kukicha*)

This is a Japanese green tea blend made from stems, stalks, and twigs. Infused with vitamins and nutrients, kukicha has six times more calcium than cow milk and two and a half times more vitamin C than oranges. Very low in caffeine, kukicha reduces the risk of certain types of cancers, fights fatigue, and helps burn fat.

To make: Add one teaspoon kukicha for every two cups of boiling water.

ROASTED BARLEY TEA

A caffeine-free, roasted grain–based infusion made from barley. Traditionally used for detoxification, roasted barley tea is a staple of the Middle East and southern Europe. A hot drink in the winter and a cool drink in the summer, it is rich in antioxidants and recognized for its many health benefits. Often used as a caffeine-free coffee substitute because it has a fuller body, similar to coffee.

To make: Add two tablespoons roasted barley to four cups of boiling water.

FERMENTED VEGETABLES

Using a variety of vegetables, 80 percent being cabbage and/or a variety of hard root vegetables (beets, turnips, carrots, sweet potatoes), which also make a great base. Get creative and try different variations of vegetables you like.

1. Start by peeling the vegetables, as the skin tends to become bitter during fermentation. Finely chop all the chosen vegetables or use a food processor. Keeping in mind that anything leafy green will turn to mush.

2. Sparingly add seasonings such as ginger, garlic, and onion. Keep in mind that fermentation increases flavor tenfold, so be mindful of overpowering the vegetables.

3. Option to add sea vegetables, such as wakame, dulse, or seaweed flakes for extra mineral and fiber nutrients.

4. Herbs can also help to add flavor and make it your own. Try basil, rosemary, sage, oregano, or thyme.

5. I recommend using a vitamin K2 starter culture packet to encourage quick fermenting and added benefits. Dissolve in water or celery juice. Note that this is optional, as cabbage will ferment on its own.

6. Once everything is in a bowl, massage the vegetables and squeeze them to release the juices. Continue to do this for a couple of minutes. *Put your positive love and intentions into the food.*

7. Add a pinch of sea salt, if desired, and put contents into a wide mouth mason jar.

8. Tightly pack the vegetables by pushing down with your fist or a wooden utensil until juices come to the top of the mixture.

9. Lastly, place a whole cabbage leave on top before placing lid on.

10. Open the jar daily to release any pressure.

11. Vegetables should be kept at room temperature for four to seven days. Then you can place in refrigerator and can keep anywhere from four to eighteen months.

MILLET MASHED POTATOES

This is a medicinal version of your regular mashed potatoes. You will be shocked at how similar, and even better, they taste.

1. Layer one cup of cauliflower, one-half cup rinsed millet, and a pinch of sea salt in a large pot,

2. Add two and a half cups of water, trying not to disturb the layers. The layering allows the flavors of the vegetables to cook up into the grain without having to stir.

3. Cover and bring to a boil.

4. Reduce heat and simmer for about forty-five minutes, or until all the liquid has been absorbed and the millet is soft.

5. Add one teaspoon of roasted sesame tahini and mash with a potato masher.

6. Serve with hemp seeds, scallion, parsley, or any other herb or condiment you desire.

BROWN RICE WITH KOMBU

Brown rice contains an ideal balance of nutrients and is a principle staple in the macrobiotic diet. Adding kombu to the soaking process allows the nutrients of the sea vegetables to be integrated into the rice. Macrobiotics believe that 50 percent or more of each meal should be centered around grains.

1. Wash well, one cup of organic brown rice, massaging the rice in the water and rinsing.

2. Cut a one-inch piece of kombu and add to rice.

3. Cover with water and soak overnight.

4. In the morning, place contents into a nabe pot (ceramic pot) and add enough water so that water is one inch over the rice.

5. Take out kombu and eat or toss into compost.

6. Bring rice to a boil, and then cover and simmer until water is gone and rice is completely cooked.

You can use the same preparation to soak legumes the night before. Some good options are lentils, mung beans, kidney beans, and white or black beans.

SOUP
Soups done right can be very filling, hearty to the soul, and healing to the body. The key is in choosing a variety of seasonal vegetables. Think outside the box and choose vegetables you don't normally use. For instance, add daikon root, fennel, or bok choy. Choose noodles for more substance, such as udon, rice noodles, or mochi. Miso soup is a traditional Japanese staple made from a variety of grains and soybeans. Rich in friendly bacteria and enzymes, miso is commonly eaten as a morning soup in a macrobiotic diet. A natural antibiotic, miso is the "chicken soup" in many Asian cultures.

MISO SOUP
Purchase good quality miso: barley miso (*mugi miso*), soybean miso (*hatcho miso*), or brown rice miso (*genmai miso*).

1. Soak a one-half inch piece of wakame in cold water for about five minutes, and then cut into small pieces.

2. Add the wakame to a pot with one cup of water and bring to a boil.

3. Meanwhile, choose two to three vegetables and cut them into little pieces. Options to try include celery, carrots, shiitake, burdock root, cabbage, onion, broccoli, cauliflower, leek, and corn.

4. Add the vegetables to the boiling broth and boil for another three to five minutes or until the vegetables are soft.

5. Dilute miso (measure one half to one level teaspoon per cup of broth) in a little bit of water.

6. Add to soup and simmer for three to five minutes on a low flame.

7. Option to add tofu, mochi, grains, or beans for a thicker soup.

8. Garnish with scallions, parsley, or dandelion leaves.

I always say "nature first" and when needing to satisfy my sweet tooth, it is no different. Look to nature first. The natural sweets of the earth contain an abundance of vitamins and nutrients that our bodies need and can satisfy any sweet tooth. Here are two of my favorite unusual versions on some yummy desserts.

BAKED APPLES

One large, organic, preferably green apple (contains less sugar), three teaspoons roasted sesame seeds, two teaspoons organic raisins, three teaspoons brown rice syrup.

1. Wash the apple and cut out the core so that the opening is about one inch in diameter and the bottom is intact.

2. Put sesame seeds and raisins in a suribachi (Japanese mortar and pestle) to grind them coarsely.

3. Put mixture into a bowl, add rice syrup, and mix together.

4. Fill the apple cavity with mixture and place on baking dish.

5. Cover and bake at 350 degrees for twenty minutes.

KANTEN

Kanten is a healthy alternative to Jell-O. It is a vegan gelatin processed from sea vegetables. One-half cup organic apple juice with a few grains of sea salt, one teaspoon agar-agar (magical seaweed with the added benefit of relieving constipation), and one-third cup fruit (apple, pear, peach, or whatever you desire).

1. Combine in a sauce pan the apple juice, sea salt, and agar-agar. Gradually stir the agar-agar until it dissolves.

2. Once dissolved, bring to a boil then reduce heat and simmer for about ten minutes.

3. Add fruit slices if you wish and mix.

4. Pour mixture into one large dish or several little ones and set aside. Once cool, place in refrigerator for forty-five minutes to an hour or until jelled.

Other Healthier Sweet Options: Honey, frozen kefir, fruit, dates, prunes, carob, coconut, smoothies, and other naturally sweet juices.

Part 2
Body

Get Moving

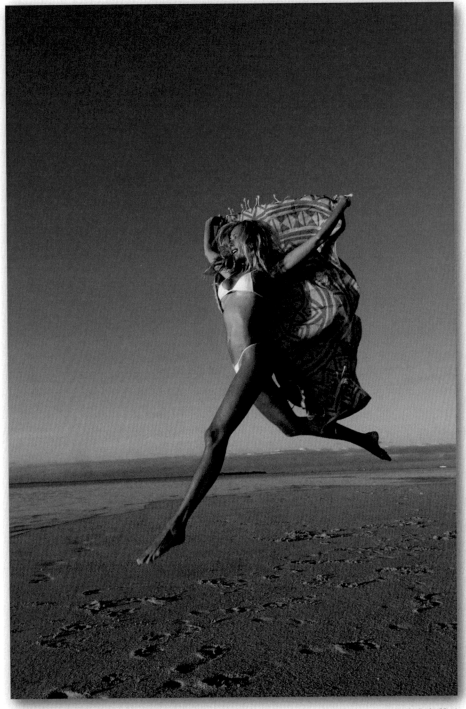

Photo by Luba Vitti

We all know that diet and exercise are the keys to optimal health, but it's not about the knowing, it's about the doing.

I often notice people talking about getting fit more than actually doing what it takes to get fit. If we put that time and energy into *just moving*, then we would most likely attain our goal. I am always striving to keep things simple, and I encourage you to do the same. So no need for the best gym membership, or one at all! Don't overthink it and let go of excuses like, "I can't go to yoga class because I can't touch my toes!" That is the whole point of going! Keep it simple and just move.

Don't know where to start? Start with *The Golden Secrets Yoga*, a sequence of exercises rooted with the foundation of different types of yoga, ballet, and physical conditioning that if practiced several times a week can help optimize your health and turn back the clock.

An easy and effective thing to keep your body and mind fit is to take ten- to twenty-minute walks outside in fresh air one to three times per day, preferably right after meals. Do not wait for your food to settle…it will digest much faster if you move!

However, avoid anything too strenuous after a meal as the body will focus on the muscles performing the exercise, leaving your digestive system to fend for itself.

TRY HIIT

HIIT (high intensity interval training) is one of the most effective ways to shed extra weight and build endurance. Unlike standard cardio, interval training offers more benefits in less time. Start with walking one minute, then running one minute, and then repeat three to five times. Eventually building up to five minutes walking and then five minutes running, repeating three to five times. Start off with short bursts, and as you build up your strength and stamina, you will spend longer periods in your intensity zone. Another option to try is, instead of focusing on the duration of time that you are in your intense zone, you can do more reps. Either way you do it, this is by far one of the most effective ways to transform your body.

Be creative at home. If you don't have weights, use your detergent bottle for weight or walk to the local market and carry your grocery bags home. Get "old-school" and do jumping jacks, jump rope, push-ups, or sit-ups. Just get your heart rate up.

CREATE A CIRCUIT TRAINING COURSE AT HOME:
Choose any four to eight exercises that work the whole body. Start by doing thirty seconds of each move and build up from there, making the repetitions longer or the movements more difficult. Rest one minute in between cycles. Repeat each cycle three to five times.

OPTIONS TO TRY:

- If you have access to stairs, run up and down them, jump squat up and down them, or do lunges up them and jog down them.

- Sit-ups (twist variation or add weights)

- Push-ups (modify on knees or do standing wall push-ups)

- Front kicks

- High knees

- Burpees

- Triceps dips

- Jump rope

- Jog in place

- Jumping jacks

- Squats

- Side plank

- Mountain climbers

- Bicycle kicks

GET THE KIDS INVOLVED
Play hopscotch, jump rope, or tag with the kids, or like a kid! Or put on your favorite music and dance. No more excuses. Just move and break a sweat!

Any kind of physical activity that helps you to break a sweat purges your body of built-up toxins and gets the job done.

LISTEN TO YOUR BODY

Some days a brisk walk will do the trick, other days, a spinning class, followed by a yoga class will be what your body desires. Listen to what your body needs each day and adjust accordingly.

If swollen or stiff joints are preventing you from moving, then you need to move even more! Regular exercise triggers endorphins that help to reduce our perception of pain, and it's also one of the most potent ways to combat inflammation in the body and prevent it. Inflammation is one of the major factors that causes us to age more rapidly.

Every synovial joint in our body has something called synovial fluid inside of it. This synovial fluid is what keeps our joints lubricated and mobile, allowing us to move. The only way to create more synovial fluid is by moving those joints! So, your movements don't have to be anything extreme, they just have to be something. They can be as simple as opening and closing your hands, or bringing your arms up and down over your head. Another great thing to do is sets of sitting in a chair and standing back up.

Remember, sometimes moving hurts, but not moving hurts more.

As we age, it is even more important that we stay mobile and stable.

The Center for Disease Control (CDC) reports that each year, one in three adults, over the age of sixty-five will fall. In order to stay steady on your feet, you need to be steady on your feet.

Physical activity is also a must for people with hypothyroidism (an underactive thyroid), a condition that can cause such fatigue and fogginess that any kind of movement can be difficult. Physical exercise can positively affect the consequences associated with hypothyroidism, such as depression and elevated cholesterol levels.

Regular exercise can help everyone boost their metabolism, help shed unwanted weight, fight fatigue, and lift up their spirits. So what are you waiting for? Get up and move!

WHAT NOT TO DO

Avoid sitting for long periods of time. If your work requires you to be at a desk for long periods of time, then switch to a standing desk. Standing desks are becoming more common due to their health benefits and people's need to be working on their computer for long periods of time.

Switching to a standing desk should be a gradual process. Start with one to two hours of standing per day and let your body gradually adapt. Be mindful to not stand in one place too long. It is important to move regularly and stretch while standing too.

Another great alternative to standard desk chairs are medicine balls (large balls designed to sit on). Medicine balls encourage movement by making it easy to bounce and stretch while at your desk.

On days that you are working long hours sitting, get up and move every twenty minutes. Walk, stretch, do some jumping jacks. Or if you work from home, step away from your desk and do another task that needs to be done to take a break from sitting.

Rule of thumb, get up and move for at least two minutes before sitting back down.

According to a study in the March 26, 2012, issue of *Archives of Internal Medicine*, researchers discovered that people who sat for eleven hours a day or more were 40 percent more likely to die, from any cause. The researchers also found the odds of dying were 15 percent higher for those who sit between eight to eleven hours a day compared to those who sit less than four hours a day.

Even if you work out for an hour a day, it will not counteract the negative side effects from sitting for long periods of time. You must get up and move throughout your day! Ideally it is recommended that you split your time between standing and sitting.

TO DO
Be mindful of your posture when sitting and standing. Focus on keeping your spine straight, as your spine's job is to keep your brain alert. Engage your core and keep your shoulders back and neck long.

Break a sweat, but don't let the workout break you. Be mindful of your energy level each day. Rest days are just as important as workout days. We do not want to stress our adrenal glands by going hard every day. Working out hard two to three times a week is plenty for your body. The other days can be moderate movement, walking, and stretching.

Remember when you don't want to move, it is often when you need to move most!

Stretch

I think stretching may be the most overlooked wellness, antiaging practice there is. Stretching is for *everybody*. It is not something that takes excellent skill or energy, and it can be modified to suit everyone's needs.

If you can breathe, you can stretch.

The best thing about stretching is its ability to continually increase your range of motion, helping you to age gracefully. I often see people in their thirties struggle to get their shoes on and I think to myself, "Wow, how are you going to be at seventy?" Stay ahead of the game and stretch every day. Yes, every day and start now!

I am not naturally flexible; I practice stretching every day.

FOLLOW MY *GOLDEN SECRETS YOGA* GUIDELINES:

- Start slow and build up to deeper stretches. There is no magic pill. As I have said, flexibility is achieved by stretching *every day*.

- When you are scheduling your workouts, take into account time to stretch. Stretch after a workout, bath, or sauna when your muscles are warm and more likely to open up.

- Find the place within the stretch where you feel change happening, but not pain. If you feel pain, then pull back. Take a deep inhale, and on the exhale, let any tension or gripping go (this includes your jaw).

- Open your mouth on the exhale when you are doing intense stretching. Release of the jaw can mimic a release in other parts of your body.

- We tend to hold onto stress and negative emotions in the body, causing us to become rigid and stiff. Every part of the body is associated with an experience in our life or something we are resisting. When we are able to connect the experience to the particular body part causing us the pain, we can replace the experience with a positive one and begin to heal and open up. *Flexible body, flexible mind.*

- Stay in the stretch for a minimum of thirty seconds so that your muscle fibers have time to release and maintain results.

- Always be mindful when coming out of a stretch in order to prevent injury. Slow and steady. This is not a time to rush.

- *If you stretch every day, you will notice each movement becomes easier.*

Get your ZZZs

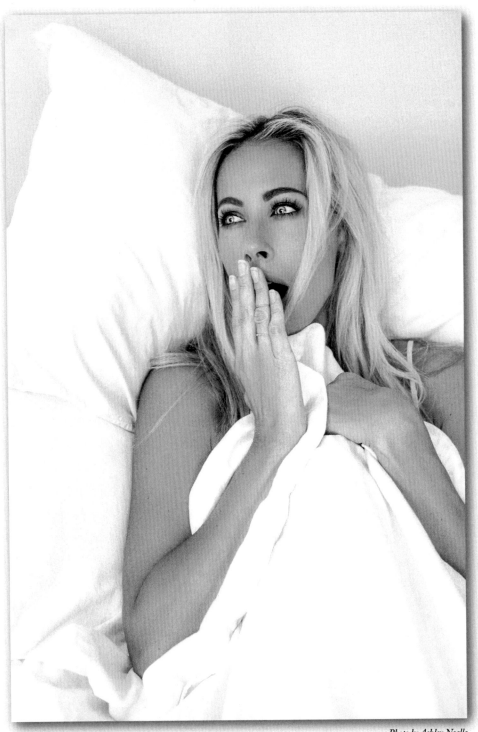

Photo by Ashley Noelle

Y ou need sleep as much as you need to breath. Not getting adequate sleep each night can weaken your immune system, slow down your metabolism, and decrease your ability to function properly.

It is ideal that adults get seven to nine hours of sleep each night in order for their bodies to have enough time to recover and get ready for the next day. Growing children, babies, and those suffering from an illness need much more. Without sufficient sleep we are susceptible to suffering from a variety of ailments and illnesses, including mood swings, lack of concentration, and poor food choices, creating even more health issues.

Whether you suffer from insomnia or just don't seem to have enough time to get adequate sleep, it is crucial to learn healthy sleep habits so that your body can function at its best.

HERE ARE SOME IDEAS TO HELP YOU GET SUFFICIENT SLEEP EACH NIGHT:

- Set a schedule and go to sleep and wake up at the same time every day, even on the weekends! Your body works best on a set schedule. When the schedule gets thrown off is when problems can occur.

- Set your alarm for your desired time and just get up! Pressing the snooze button to get an extra fifteen minutes of sleep actually does more harm than good. Going back into a deep sleep disturbs your natural sleep rhythms, which may make it more difficult to get up.

- Keep your bedroom sacred and free from clutter, work stuff, or anything that isn't supposed to be in the bedroom. Your bedroom should be inviting and calming, so be mindful of the colors you choose for your bedroom. Muted, soft, natural colors are the best for a bedroom. Bright, igniting colors tend to keep the brain active and could keep you up.

- Invest in a good mattress, sheets, and pillows that make you want to get into bed. As humans, we spend a third of our lives sleeping so you should absolutely love where you are spending all that time.

- Refrain from drinking caffeine past breakfast or early lunch. It is good to keep in mind that decaffeinated coffee has small traces of caffeine in it, so after early afternoon, avoid it as well.

- Increase your exposure to light during the day. Light exposure plays a key role in telling us when to be awake and when to sleep. So during the day, let the light into your house or go outside for a walk.

- On the contrary, refrain from being exposed to too much artificial light twenty minutes prior to bedtime. This includes watching television, working on your computer, or being on your smartphone. The light from these devices stimulates serotonin in the body, which keeps us awake. Being in complete darkness tells our bodies that it is time for melatonin to be released.

- Get your workout in. Lack of exercise can contribute to poor sleep. However, intense exercise too close to bedtime can increase your chances of staying up, so it is best to sweat it out during the day.

- Give yourself adequate time to decompress and start winding down prior to your actual bedtime. If you are out to dinner, have a chamomile tea with dessert or as dessert. The calming chamomile herbs will help you release the stresses from the day, preparing you for a peaceful night sleep.

- Create healthy nighttime rituals while you are preparing for bed. Spend some time washing the day away by cleaning your face, flossing, brushing your teeth, and putting your bedtime remedies on your skin. Maybe saying some positive affirmations to yourself, acknowledging the good day you had. Creating positive associations with bedtime as a time for you to let the day go and let your body regenerate.

- Keep a diary, and just before bed either review your day or write an intention for your next day. After you are done writing, let go of both today and tomorrow's plans. Then when you get to thirty days take a night off to read what you wrote.

- Make positive life changes before reaching for sleeping pills. I believe the benefits of minor life changes to achieve adequate sleep far outweighs the convenience and negative side effects of sleeping pills.

- Don't count sheep, count your blessings. Using the alphabet, find something you are grateful for that starts with the letter A and continue all the way through Z, finding a blessing with each letter. You can do this every night in your bed silently or out loud. It encourages healthy bedtime rituals of gratitude, and it also makes a great bedtime practice for children who don't want to go to sleep.

NATURAL REMEDIES FOR A MORE RESTFUL SLEEP:

- **Melatonin:** Melatonin is produced from serotonin when exposure to light decreases at night. Due to aging, jet lag, or sleep disorders, some people can have low levels of melatonin. Supplementing it may improve quality of sleep and morning alertness.

- **"Rescue Remedy" sleep formula**: a natural flower remedy that calms your restless mind to relieve occasional sleeplessness.

- **Chamomile tea:** Roman chamomile tea has been used for centuries to calm and aid in relieving sleeping problems.

- **Calcium and magnesium**: two essential minerals for optimal health. Taking them together allows your body to absorb them properly. A deficiency in either can cause sleep disturbances, so supplementing at night can help you reach a deeper level of sleep.

- **Herbs:** such as ashwagandha, ginkgo biloba, reishi mushroom, valerian root, and Siberian ginseng. Always consult your doctor before starting any new remedy, herbal or otherwise.

- **Aromatherapy:** Try a couple of drops of lavender, chamomile, vetiver, valerian, marjoram, neroli, or clary sage oil in a warm bath prior to bed, on your pillow, or massaged into the soles of your feet to connect to all the systems of the body and help you relax.

- **Tryptophan:** Studies show that the lack of the essential amino acid tryptophan could be responsible for insomnia and even depression. Tryptophan is necessary for the production of serotonin, and if serotonin is deficient, it could cause you to lose sleep as well as impair your memory and concentration. Some plant-based food sources of tryptophan include spirulina, nuts, flaxseeds, chai seeds, pumpkin seeds, sesame seeds (or tahini), and beans.

Sleep is the best meditation.

—The Dalai Lama

Toxin-free

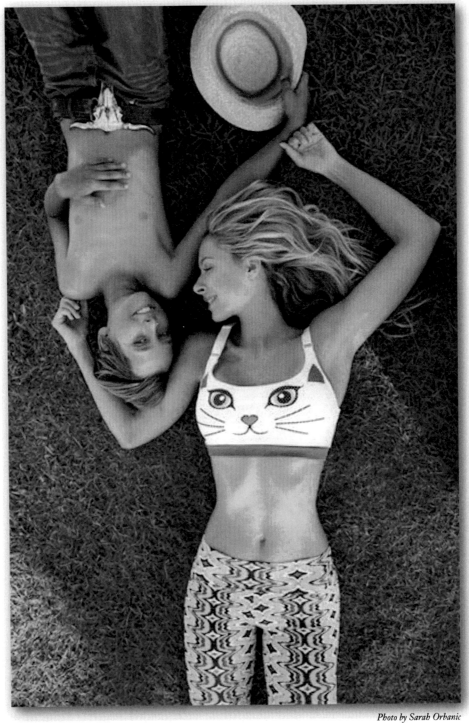

Photo by Sarah Orbanic

These days it is nearly impossible to be free of all toxins. Toxins are everywhere: in our food, in the air, and in most consumer and cleaning products. Even if you stayed home to avoid toxins, you may be better off going outside, because most toxins are actually found in our own homes.

Studies show that the risk of chronic illness and even cancer is higher for people who are stay-at-home parents or for those who spend a lot of time indoors.

I believe that the majority of mass advertising tries to convince us that consumer cleaning products make our homes clean and safe, when really we are overloading our bodies with more toxins! Empower yourself and stay away from toxic home and personal products. We do have a choice in this. Choose to support companies and brands that encourage health for yourself, your family, and the environment.

HOW TO AVOID TOXINS:

- Natural cleaning products can be made from products you already have at home. For example, use apple cider vinegar, baking soda, and essential oils such as tea tree oil and lavender for disinfecting. Cedarwood and rosemary oils are good for polishing wood and furniture. Thieves oil (a blend of clove, cinnamon bark, rosemary, lemon, and eucalyptus) is a great oil to use as an air mist in the home anytime, but it is especially helpful when someone has been ill as it helps clean the air. Lemongrass oil does wonders to clean toilets, garbage cans, and garbage disposals.

- Start a no-shoe policy. Not only will you have to clean your house less frequently, but you will also keep more harmful toxins out of your home. *Scientists say that shoes, on average, carry 421,000 units of bacteria, including E coli and herbicides.*

- Be mindful of the clothes you purchase and, when possible, buy natural and organic fabrics. Support clothing lines that are eco-friendly and represent fashion in a sustainable way.

- To help minimize computer radiation, place a bowl of charcoal and distilled water on the left side of your computer and place a green plant on the right. Replace both every two to three months.

- Green plants with large leaves naturally help keep the air in your house clean. Ideally place one plant in each room. Some of the best green plants include philodendron, golden pathos, Ficus, areca palm, aloe vera, and Boston fern.

- The amount of fire retardant and chemicals that mattresses are doused in is often a big secret. We spend more than a third of our lives in our bed, so be sure your mattress is chemical-free and toxin-free.

Of the chemicals found in homes, 150 have been linked to allergies, birth defects, cancer, and psychological abnormalities.

—CONSUMER PRODUCT SAFETY COMMISSION (2007)

NATURAL CLEANING RECIPES

ALL-PURPOSE CLEANER
Equal parts white vinegar and warm water, juice from half a lemon, and several drops of tea tree oil or essential oil of your choice. Pour into a spray bottle for easy cleaning. Great for windows and mirrors, too. *Vinegar naturally kills mold, germs, and bacteria.*

HEAVY-DUTY BATHROOM CLEANER
One tablespoon of Castile soap, one tablespoon of baking soda, several drops of tea tree oil, and warm water. Great for cleaning toilets, sinks, tubs, and tiles. *The baking soda neutralizes odors and is a natural scrubbing agent. Tea tree oil is effective against bacteria and viruses.*

FURNITURE POLISH
Choose a natural oil base, such as olive or almond oil. Add several drops of cedarwood, rosemary, or orange essential oil and mix with warm water.

ULTIMATE FLOOR CLEANER
In a bucket, add one cup of white vinegar, one tablespoon of Castile soap, one cup of baking soda, and fifteen to twenty drops of geranium or lavender essential oil or scent of your choice. Fill the rest of the bucket with hot water and mop.

THE SPA EXPERIENCE AT HOME
Place a couple drops of eucalyptus essential oil into the corners of your shower for an invigorating experience. The hot water will diffuse the oil into the bathroom creating a healthy steam, all while naturally cleaning the shower. *Be careful not to put the oil where your standing as it can create a slippery situation.*

Everything we put into and onto our bodies matters. It only takes twenty-six seconds for chemicals and toxins from personal care products to enter our bloodstream. So we need to be mindful of the beauty and skin care products we choose. Buy organic, natural, and toxin-free products. As an extra benefit, most of these health conscious products are cruelty-free and environmentally conscious.

There is one product that has had much controversy, yet many people still choose to use it every single day and believe in the benefits over the negative side effects: I am talking about fluoride toothpaste.

Despite what many believe, fluoride is not approved by the FDA for the prevention of cavities.

Through mass media, we are tricked into believing that without fluoride all of our teeth would decay quickly. This is simply not true and in the meantime, we may be seriously affecting our bodies with the toxic effects of fluoride.

According to data from Harvard University, fluoride exposure showed damaging effects on neurological and cognitive development in children. Fluoride can cause arthritis, dementia, severe eye problems, and impaired thyroid function. And if that isn't enough, fluoride actually causes dental fluorosis and decay in the tooth enamel. Putting you right back in the dental chair!

Have you ever looked at the label of your fluoride toothpaste? The label warns that if you swallow a quarter-milligram of fluoride that you should immediately contact poison control.

In 2015 the US Department of Health and Human Services lowered the allowable levels of fluoride in water to 0.7 milligrams per liter of water, from its previous 1.2 milligrams. The reasons given for that change were that we now get fluoride from many other resources, including toothpastes and mouthwashes.

You don't need fluoride to have a beautiful smile. Have you ever seen the beautiful smiles of the indigenous people of Africa, or other remote areas of the world that don't have access to fluoride? I believe these people have some of the most beautiful smiles in the world. Granted they are not eating all the sugary and artificial foods that we have access to either, but that too should be taken into account when desiring a beautiful smile.

We have to remember that at one time doctors recommended cocaine toothache drops and morphine soothing syrup.

As with anything, being educated, mindful, and listening to your own inner wisdom are some of the most powerful tools you have.

We must remain open and clear about the source of our ideas and information because many times the studies we base our viewpoints on are paid for by the companies benefiting from the outcomes.

There are many natural ways to achieve a healthy, beautiful smile without compromising our health.

HERE ARE SOME HEALTHY ALTERNATIVES TO FLUORIDE THAT REALLY GET TO THE ROOT OF THE PROBLEM AND CAN MAKE YOU HEALTHIER:

BAKING SODA, SEA SALT, PEPPERMINT OR TEA TREE ESSENTIAL OIL

Make your own paste by mixing the following into a glass jar: two-thirds cup baking soda, a large pinch of sea salt, five to ten drops of organic peppermint or tea tree essential oil. Mix until it reaches the consistency of toothpaste.

FLOSS REGULARLY

Preferably after each meal, but at least every evening before bed. Water picks are a must for people who have a difficult time flossing.

ORAL PULLING RINSE

An Ayurveda practice that uses oils to pull out toxins from the mouth and prevent these toxins from getting to the rest of your body. Vigorously swish, push, and pull oil throughout your entire mouth for up to twenty minutes. You can use sesame, safflower, argon, or coconut oil, all of which you may already have in your kitchen cupboard. For extra benefit, add an essential oil of your liking, for example, clove, tea tree, or peppermint. Do not gargle with oral pulling rinse.

GARGLES AND MOUTHWASH

Make your own natural mouthwash and gargles with a couple drops of essential oil. Fennel and thyme essential oils are helpful in the treatment of bad breath, mouth sores or ulcers, gum infections, and sore throats. Add a couple of drops of oil to a glass of warm water and gargle or swish in your mouth for several seconds.

SEAWEED TOOTHPASTE

Although raw, unheated seaweed might not be your favorite thing to brush with, studies show that seaweed produces enzymes that may be able to remove the microbes in dental plaque, which is made up of decaying bacteria that causes damage in the mouth. Seaweed toothpaste is available at many local health food stores.

TONGUE CLEANER

Regularly using a tongue cleaner can prevent plaque and bacteria from getting into your teeth and your body. It also reduces bad breath and improves your taste buds. After brushing, put the tongue cleaner as far back on your tongue as you can and scrape forward to the tip of your tongue. Rinse the cleaner and continue one or two more times until there is no longer any residue left on the tongue cleaner when you scrape it.

COCONUT OIL

Coconut oil contains powerful microbes that destroy viruses and bacteria. Add baking soda to the coconut oil and you have a natural bacteria fighting, whitening toothpaste. It is also great for oral pulling.

FENNEL TEA

Gargle with fennel tea to freshen breath and to heal infected gums and sore throats.

CLOVE OIL

Dilute a couple drops of clove oil into a clean bowl of water. Soak a clean cloth in the water. Ring out the excess water and then put into the freezer until frozen. The cold compress can be used for any soreness in the mouth, toothache, or baby teething. The clove oil will naturally numb the discomfort.

A smile is the best thing you will ever wear.

External Remedies

Did you know that our skin is our largest organ? Our bodies absorb everything we put onto it through our pores. The skin is also the primary organ of elimination so it is important that we take great care of it by incorporating healthy daily rituals. If you eat organically and then apply toxins to your skin, you are doing a disservice to your body.

BODY SCRUBBING

Body scrubbing is one of the easiest ways to detox the body of unwanted pollutants. You are already in the shower cleaning yourself, so just give yourself a little more TLC while you are in there. The heat from the shower opens up the pores, and the scrubbing creates blood circulation, removes dead skin cells, and releases toxins that the body has absorbed.

Stimulating your body in this way every day not only discharges and helps flush your body of toxins, but it also flushes unwanted fat and cellulite. Daily body scrubbing wipes away the grime of daily living and removes environmental toxins.

While you sleep, the body excels in its regenerative abilities. By adding body scrubbing to your daily routine, your body will detoxify and renew more efficiently while you sleep.

Some people are afraid that if they scrub everyday they will lose their tan, but the effect of scrubbing is quite the contrary. After establishing a habit of scrubbing, your skin will create its own natural golden glow.

STEPS FOR BODY SCRUBBING:

1. While taking a shower, let your body heat up so that your pores are open.

2. Use a rough hand mitt or a washcloth. I prefer to use a rough hand mitt as opposed to a soft loofah.

3. Turn the shower off (and keep the door closed so that the heat stays in the bathroom).

4. Begin vigorously scrubbing your body in circular motions, from the hands to the heart and from the feet to the heart. Scrub with enough force to create a pinkish/red tone to the skin. This pinkish/red tone is a good sign. It means that your blood is moving.

5. Once complete, quickly rinse yourself off and dry off completely. For added benefit, rinse with cold water to close your pores.

DAIKON HIP BATH

Daikon hip baths aid in removing toxins and excess oils from the body as well as burning excess fat, therefore helping with any skin issues as well as being great for women's reproductive organs.

1. Use freshly dried daikon leaves. If daikon is hard to find, you can use turnip leaves or arame seaweed (kelp).

2. Place about four or five bunches into a large pot of water (four to five quarts) and bring to a boil.

3. Cover and simmer until the water turns brown.

4. Add one cup of sea salt and stir well to help dissolve.

5. Strain liquid into a hot bath so that water is waist high when sitting in the tub.

6. Sit in the tub and cover your upper body with a towel to induce perspiration.

7. Stay in the bath for ten to twenty minutes, until your hip area becomes very red.

8. Be careful getting out as you may be a little light-headed.

9. Promptly dry off and dress appropriately to keep your body warm.

This bath is best done before bed, at least one hour after eating, and it can be done up to two times per week. It is not recommended during menstruation or if you're pregnant or nursing.

HOT/COLD THERAPY

Heat increases perspiration and therefore aids in removing toxins, and cold engages the healing response. Ideally it is best to go from a hot sauna to a cold shower. Most of us do not have a sauna at our disposal, but some of us may have a separate shower and bath. Enabling you to go from a hot bath to a cold shower.

1. The hot phase should get you warm enough to sweat but not deliriously hot.

2. The cold phase should not bring about shivers but should cool you down.

3. Generally, three cycles back to back. Starting with hot.

4. The stronger the immune system, the more resistance to the extremes you will be. Staying in the heat for a prolonged time can weaken you, so be wise and gentle.

5. Gauge the time and temperatures according to your health and needs.

GINGER SCRUB

Ginger body scrubs create circulation, promote clear skin, help discharge accumulated fat, open up skin pores to help elimination of toxins, and stimulate overall health and well-being.

1. Boil several cups of water on the stove.

2. Grate ginger and wrap into a cheesecloth. Squeeze juice into boiling water.

3. Remove from stove and let cool.

4. With a loofah, or preferably a rough hand mitt, stand in the shower or bath with your ginger water in a bowl and begin scrubbing with the shower off.

5. Always scrub toward your heart and don't forget in between your fingers and toes, behind your ears, the undersides of your hands, and the soles of your feet. Scrub vigorously to get the blood flowing. Your skin should become pink or slightly red.

6. When you are done scrubbing your entire body, quickly rinse off and put a robe on to keep the heat in.

Best done separate from shower or bath, either before or after, and prior to bed. Can be done up to two times per week.

CABBAGE COMPRESS

Carefully peel two cabbage leafs from a cabbage and apply to sore joints or anywhere on the body that has inflammation. Best done at bedtime, as you are lying still and the leaves can be on you for a longer period of time.

Mastitis, a common ailment of breastfeeding mothers, is when a milk duct becomes clogged, causing it to become infected, engorged, and painful. An old midwifery cure is to place a cabbage leaf inside the mother's bra overnight. I have personally done this myself and know many others that, too, have been miraculously cured by a cabbage leaf.

DRY BRUSHING
Dry brushing massage essentially does the same thing as body scrubbing but it is done prior to showering, removing dead skin cells so that new ones can be formed. Dry brushing also helps the body breathe, absorb oxygen, and throw off toxins. The increased circulation also brings blood to the skin's surface, tightening it and giving it a natural golden glow, helping you to look years younger.

1. Before you shower, use a natural bristle brush (found at a health food store) or a natural loofah or sponge. Start at your feet moving upward toward your torso. Always move toward your heart and brush your entire body, not forgetting the nooks and crannies, including between the toes and behind the ears.

2. Add a couple drops of your favorite essential oil to your brush for an added health benefit and soothing experience. Always dilute oils before putting them directly on skin. Some suggested oils are lavender and chamomile.

DO-IN SELF MASSAGE
Do-in is a self-applied energy to revitalize and energize your body and mind, the epitome of giving yourself some love. It is amazing what a couple minutes of massaging, rubbing, and targeting trigger points can do. Below is one variation that takes less than three minutes; best practiced in the morning to get things moving.

1. With relaxed wrists and fingers, begin to tap the head from the corner of the eyebrows, over the head to the base of the skull. Repeat as many times as needed.

2. Then move on to the cheekbones, jaw, and side of the neck.

3. Holding onto one elbow across your body tap the opposite shoulder. Repeat on other side.

4. With loose wrists you can tap your chest (Tarzan style) and then down the inside of one arm and up the outside. Repeat on the other side.

5. Begin to brush the body from your chest to your abdomen in a downward motion.

6. Then with both hands on the belly, make circular motions in one direction (about three times), and then reverse direction.

7. Then if your shoulders allow, reach your hands back behind you and try to tap underneath the shoulder blades and down to the kidneys, back of the pelvis, and gluteus muscles.

8. Continue down the outsides of the legs and up the insides of the legs.

9. Lastly brush yourself off from the feet to the top of the head to complete your exercise.

At any time throughout the massage, you can pause and feel the warmth (energy) of your hands onto your body, focusing on any area that needs extra attention.

BELLY RUBS

Daily belly massages can aid in proper elimination, ease digestive discomfort, and sooth the entire body. Best done on an empty stomach prior to bedtime to encourage proper elimination upon waking up.

1. Thoroughly lubricate your entire belly with an organic oil. You can even use organic olive or coconut oil that you have in your kitchen.

2. Going counterclockwise, begin to deeply massage the belly, feeling for any gas or air bubbles. Encourage any air to move downward.

3. As you massage, focus on your breath, letting go of any gripping on the exhale.

4. Continue for as long as it feels comfortable.

   Some of the best medicine in the world is creating daily, healthy rituals of self-love.

Part 3
Practice

The Golden Secrets Yoga

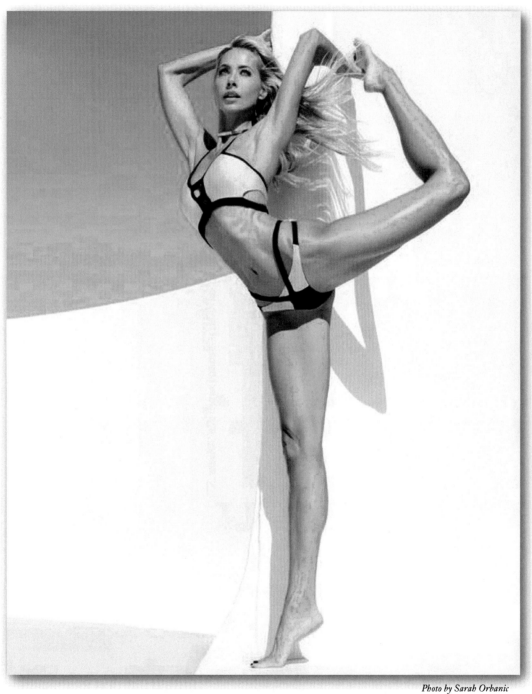

Photo by Sarah Orbanic

I created a particular set of exercises that you can do at home to help you become strong, fit, and confident, and age with grace. Rooted in the foundation of different types of yoga, ballet, and physical conditioning, this series, if practiced several times a week, will help you feel your best and turn back the clock.

Every move has a purpose, a breath, and a focus point. Growing up as a ballerina, for years I spent hours in the dance studio training. Physically it allowed me a graceful transition into yoga, but the awareness of breath and mindfulness in connection with the body's movements was a whole new world—a world that I was craving and one that felt right at home. Through years of experience with the body and movement, along with the philosophy of yoga, I wanted to develop and share a sequence for everyone that had purpose and positive effects on one's health.

- Strengthen your core and learn how to tap into your powerhouse.

- Create flexibility to keep you agile and open-minded. As we age we can become rigid, not only in our bodies but in our minds.

- Build strength to develop and maintain your equilibrium so that you will have a solid foundation of balance.

- Activate the seven chakras that stimulate all the glands of your endocrine system, which are responsible for the proper function of all your organs and, in turn, positively affect your overall health and keep you looking young and beautiful.

OTHER BENEFITS OF THE GOLDEN SECRETS YOGA:

- Leads to feelings of healing, rejuvenation, and empowerment.

- Increases energy and stamina.

- Improves brain function (clarity) and coordination.

- Improves breathing to achieve a longer life.

- Strengthens muscles, removing common aches and pains.

- Promotes deep relaxation and REM sleep.

- Detoxifies and aids in regular elimination.

- Reduces stress and removes patterns that create it.

- Reduces cellulite and tightens skin elasticity.

- Firms and tones legs and arms, creating long and lean muscles.

- Helps you to feel confident and sexy.

- Embodies ancient secrets proven to enhance one's quality of life.

Ideally, practice the Golden Secrets of Yoga three times a week, alternating with walking, hiking, or your other fitness regimens, and remember ALWAYS take the stairs.
For the goddesses: I believe in allowing your body time to rest on the first day of your moon cycle (menstrual cycle). However, do what feels right for you.
Also, use these three tools when your mind starts to wander and the exercise or pose becomes challenging:

BREATH
Shallow breathing is a sign of a lack of endurance, patience, and health. The first lesson in health is to breathe deeply. The breath links the physical body to the mind and links the mind to the life force (*prana*).

Pranayama is the process by which the vital life force is brought under conscious control to gradually reduce afflictions, calm the mind, rejuvenate the body, and initiate the awakening of higher states of consciousness.

The most common controlled breathing in yoga is called *ujjayi pranayama*, or "victorious breath." By controlling the breath, we are able to control other functions of the body. The breath is both voluntary and involuntary, so when we choose to consciously breath we generate more oxygen for the body. As we age we lose up to 30 percent of our vital lung capacity. With a regular yoga practice you can reverse this and open the body up to create more freedom for breath and bring oxygen to every cell in your body.

Begin by taking a normal inhalation and normal exhalation through the mouth, then start to bring awareness to the back of your throat. On your next exhale, begin to slightly constrict the passage of air to tone the back of the throat. Imagine you are trying to fog up a mirror. You should hear a soft hissing sound (think Darth Vader). Once you are comfortable, begin to apply this same contraction of the throat to the inhales. This is created by softly pressing your tongue to the roof of your mouth. When you are able to create this contraction for both the inhale and exhale, close the mouth and begin breathing through the nose. The breath should be audible to yourself and the people on either side of you. Once you feel comfortable, start to apply this breath to the sequence.

Deeply exhale through the mouth when necessary, using it as a release to clear out and let go. Be mindful that letting energy out of the mouth is a giving away of energy, only to be practiced when the mind is set on releasing something.

Try to maintain an even inhale and exhale, having them be the same length of time. Listen to where your breath is stagnant and focus your energy there to smooth out any congestion. Each inhalation and exhalation should be long, full, deep, and controlled.

Create your own dance to your own breath. It is always there for you to come back to.

I truly believe maintaining a steady breath is that of a truly advanced student. When the breath is calm and steady, the mind and body will follow.

If you just focused on your breath for one hour, you would feel as good or better as you would after a physical workout. As you become more in tune with your quality of breath on the mat, your breath will become your most valued tool off the mat.
The way we breathe matters, and depending on our needs, we can hone in on certain breath exercises to aid us in our practice and overall well-being. Pranayama techniques can be practiced alone, before or after your sequence and during your practice, to bring awareness internally and ease the mind.

> *As a healer, the first thing to tell every patient is to breathe deeply. Shallow breathing means no endurance, no patience.*
>
> —*Yogi Bhajan*

INTENTION
Set an intention for your practice each given day. This is a way to check in with yourself and see what it is that you need that day. The practice itself remains the same but what you get out of it and need from it changes every time you do it. Some days you will focus on settling your mind for clarity and other days you will focus on building strength for courage. There are no rules for what your intention can and cannot be, just what you desire to attain by the end of your practice.

You can choose a word or a feeling, such as clarity, love, happiness, focus, release—any word or sound that brings an associated feeling for you that can help you get the most out of your practice.

Much of the work is about breaking old patterns that no longer or have never served you and making new intentions and positive agreements with yourself. This is the most important daily practice.

The physical practice is repetitive and consistent, but the lesson itself changes daily.

FOCUSED GAZE (*Drishti*)

Through your practice you will develop focus and attention—attention of your breath, your body's messages, vital energies, and the quality of your practice. It is through being attentive that you learn where to focus.

Different exercises and poses call for different focus points. Generally speaking, looking down is more calming and relaxing, looking up is more energizing and opening. Other common gazes are at the navel, the toes, the tip of the nose, the third eye, and in twists looking as far as you can from the corners of your eyes; each encourages where you intend to go. A steady gaze right in view of eyeline is what is most common to maintain balance and develop core strength. Once you have developed that, then you can move on to looking up when it feels right.

Note: Your body will go where you look, so if you look down in standing poses you just might end up there!

> *Samskara saksat karanat purvajati jnanam. (Through sustained focus and meditation on our patterns, habits, and conditioning, we gain knowledge and understanding of our past and how we can change the patterns that aren't serving us to live more freely and fully.)*
>
> —*Yoga Sutra III.18*

YOUR PRACTICE:

- Your practice (yoga) is a tool to make your unconscious patterns conscious.

- Remember, when you don't want to do it, is often when you need to do it most.

- Go at your own pace. Start slow and add poses as you feel comfortable. Start with two to three of the first exercises listed and repeat those as many days as needed before you add more. It is not about being perfect; it is about being consistent.

- Focus on allowing your body to open up on its own time and be present in the moment. If your mind is primarily on the end goal, the gap between where you are and where you want to be can bring tension in the body that can hinder your progress.

- Most of the real limits that we confront in yoga live in our mind, not our body.

- Begin with the foundation of each pose and build up from there. The foundation is what is in contact with the floor.

- Root to rebound. Every pose has an applied downward force that creates a direct reaction upward. Applying this principle into every pose will help to create length and strength in your body with ease.

- It is best to practice on an empty stomach to reap the full benefits of this practice, so practice earlier in the day or at least one hour after a meal.

- If not stated, do each exercise for thirty seconds and you can build from there, doing what feels right to you. It is not about the number of repetitions you can do; it is about being mindful, releasing old patterns, and building long, lean muscles. In order to do this, *slower is better.*

- For stretching exercises stay in each stretch for a minimum of thirty seconds but stay as long as you like. You should feel a sensation while you stretch but never pain. If you feel pain, then pull back. It is not uncommon to have emotions arise while stretching. Acknowledge them, breath into them and let them go. An ample amount of time in each stretch will create better and quicker results. Always be mindful when coming out of a stretch. Take your time.

- Always come back to your breath, your intention, and your focus. These are your three tools that you have in your toolbox when the mind begins to wander or a pose (*asana*) becomes challenging.

The Sequence

CAT/COW

Start on your hands and knees, in a tabletop position. Have your wrists directly under your shoulders and your knees directly underneath your hips. Firmly press all ten fingers into the mat, paying special attention in between your thumb and index fingers. On an inhale, arch your back and look up so that your tailbone, chest, and head are to the sky. On an exhale, round your back by bringing your naval to your spine and your chin to your chest. Focus on having your movement be in synch with your breath. Do three to five rounds and then come back to a neutral spine before moving on.

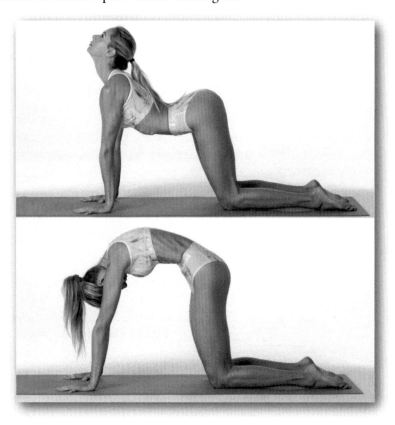

CHILD'S POSE (*Balasana*)

Bring your big toes together and sit back into your heels. If you feel any tension in your knees, you can sit on a blanket by placing it between your calves and hamstrings. As you sit into your heels, stretch your arms forward in front of you and peek up at your hands to be sure that your wrists are in line with the front edge of the mat. Press all ten fingers into the mat so much so that the forearms come up off the floor (this is the foundation to build on for future poses). Let your forehead come down onto the mat and elongate through both sides of the body evenly. Now bring your arms alongside your body, palms facing up. This is a relaxing pose should you ever get tired or dizzy and need a rest. Come to child's pose for several breaths.

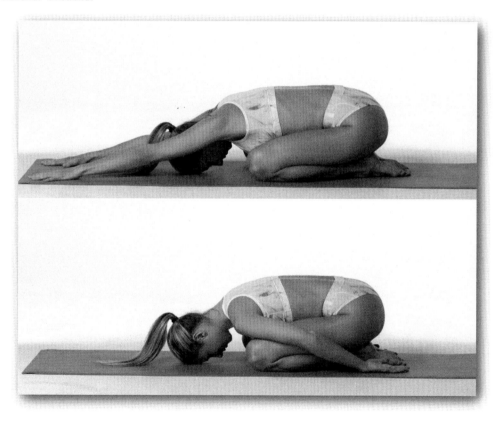

LEG/BOOTY LIFTS

Come back up onto your hands and knees, in tabletop position. Bend your right leg and flex your foot as if you are making an imprint of your foot onto the ceiling. Ideally try to start with your knee in line with your bum and pulse up from there. You can always come down onto your forearms to modify and help get your leg up higher. Begin slow and steady pulses for thirty seconds, then pause at the top and hold for ten seconds. Keep your leg where it is and open it up to the side, then lower the knee to meet the left knee. Maintain both arms equally by pressing all ten fingers into the ground. Keep your neck long and release your sit bones to the back of the room. Continue for thirty seconds. Lastly, cross the right knee over the left and then straighten it out to the side, extending all the way through the foot. Continue for thirty seconds and then repeat on the other side.

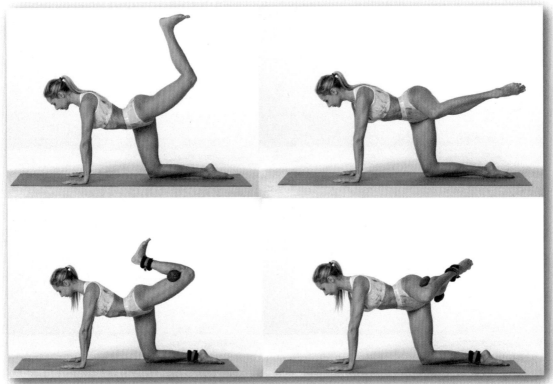

For a more advanced move, place a hand weight at the back of your knee and squeeze it tight. Also add ankle weights as well or an elastic band around the ankles for further resistance. Always add more time if it begins to get easy.

DOWNWARD-FACING DOG (*Adho Mukha Svanasana*)

Hands and feet shoulder and hip-width apart. Peek up at your hands and make sure that your wrists are straight or in line with the front edge of your mat. Press all ten fingers into the mat, especially between your thumb and index fingers. With both arms straight, but not hyperextended, rotate your outer arms toward your ears and draw your shoulder blades onto your back. Relax your head and gaze between your feet. Keep both legs straight and active. Firm your quadriceps to your hamstrings, your shins to your calves, and your heels to the ground. Once you have walked through your body and have the correct alignment, stay for three to five breaths. When you are ready to come out, slowly make your way to child's pose before standing up. At first this pose can be very challenging, but with regular practice, it will become a resting pose.

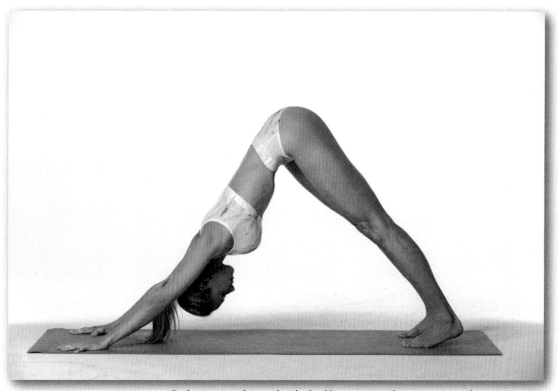

For beginners or those with tight shoulders, you can widen your arms as wide as your mat. You can also widen your legs and keep a slight bend in your knees for tight hamstrings.

HALF SUN SALUTATIONS (*Vinyasa Flow*)

Start standing, with your feet together, big toes and heels touching. Open through your chest and draw your navel up and in, draw your tailbone down, and bring your shoulders away from your ears. With an inhale, bring your arms up over your head and gaze up toward your hands, if the neck permits. Exhale as you dive forward with a flat back toward your feet. If your hamstrings are tight, widen your feet slightly and keep a small bend in the legs. Place your hands where you feel comfortable, for beginners this will be higher up on the leg, either below or above the knees, and for the more advanced the hands will be in line with the toes. With an inhale, come up to a flat back, trying to create a straight line from the tailbone to the crown of the head. For beginners the hands will again be higher up on the legs, and for advanced the hands will be in line with your toes. Exhale fold forward again, letting the belly rise in and up as you forward bend. Firm your legs and feet, and with an inhale rise all the way up with a flat back and bring your arms up over head, looking up if it feels comfortable, and then bring all that energy into your heart, ending with your hands in prayer at your chest.

Repeat three to five cycles. Focusing on one breath per movement.

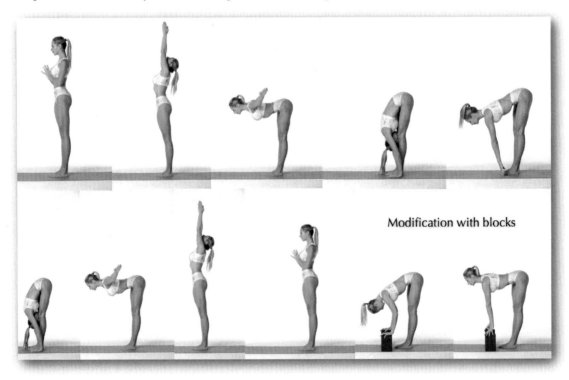

Modification with blocks

FULL SUN SALUTATIONS

After you feel comfortable with half sun salutations, or for more advanced students, you can move onto a full vinyasa flow.

Begin just as you would a half sun salutation but instead of coming back up to stand after making a flat back, on an exhale bend your knees deep so that you can get your palms flat on the floor, then step back into plank (the top of a push-up position) or for advanced, jump to *chaturanga dandasana*. If you are stepping back into plank, once there, press all ten fingers into the ground, lift up through your navel and push back into your heels so that you use your entire body to hold you up. Lower your knees to the ground to modify. Exhale and lower halfway into *chaturanga dandasana* by hugging your elbows in toward the sides of your body, making a ninety-degree angle with your arms. From here, on an inhale, you can lower all the way onto your belly and do a low cobra (*bhujangasana*) by untucking your feet and pressing all ten toes into the mat, hug your elbows in, and lift your chest off the ground, keeping your neck long. Or you can roll over your toes and come into an upward-facing dog pose (*urdhva mukha svanasana*) Straighten your arms and legs, pressing all ten toes and fingers into the ground, draw your tailbone down and lift your chest up toward the ceiling, letting your head follow if it permits. Exhale, lift the navel to the spine, roll up and over your toes to downward-facing dog. Focus your gaze between your feet and take three to five breaths. On an inhale come high onto your toes, bend your knees, and at the end of your exhale, look between your hands and step the right foot then the left foot between your hands (or jump for advanced). Inhale, lengthen the spine, creating a flat back, and exhale fold forward over your legs. Inhale, bring the arms up and over your head, coming all the way to standing and bringing all that energy back into your heart with your hands at prayer.

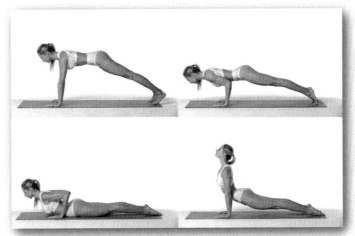

For the more advanced, add push-ups with each vinyasa and/or float up to handstand on the jump back and at the top.

Repeat three to five cycles.

TREE POSE (*Vrksasana*)

Plant your left foot (supporting leg) into the ground, with the foot pointing straight ahead. Spread the toes and press all four corners of the foot into the mat. Bring your right foot high into your inner left thigh or below the knee at your calf. Press your foot into your inner thigh by firming your standing leg, creating a resistance that will help you maintain balance. Rotate your knee to the side by drawing your tailbone down, creating an external rotation with your bent leg. Bring your hands to prayer at your heart or reach your arms up to the sky. Find something to focus on that is straight ahead. For the more advanced, try looking up toward the sky. Stay for a couple of breaths, then as graceful as you came into it, come out of it. Repeat on the other leg.

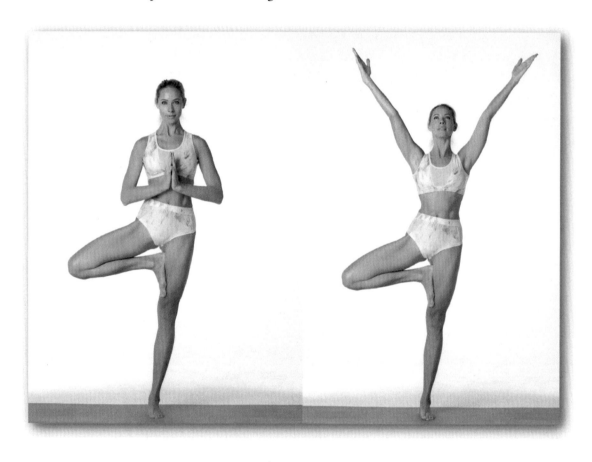

SPINNING

Arms extended out at your sides. Find a focus point to spot at the wall. As you spin clockwise, turn your head around trying to maintain focus with an eye-level focal point on the wall (spotting). Spotting is necessary for you to maintain your balance. Begin slow and make sure you have enough space to spin. It is not uncommon to feel dizzy at first. With practice this will dissipate and help you maintain your equilibrium. However, if you feel extremely dizzy, step back and modify your practice.

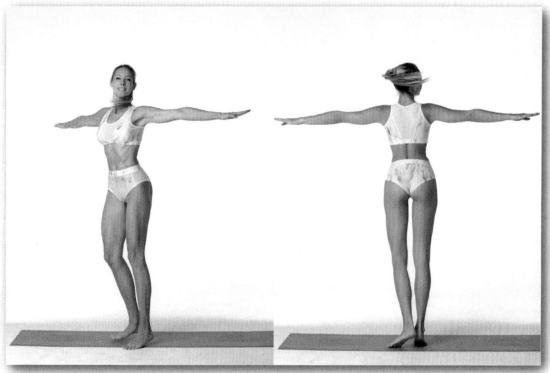

Start by spinning twice each direction and build up to eight times each direction.

JUMPING IN PLACE

Start with your heels together and your toes turned slightly out so that your knees are directly over your toes. Round your arms so that your hands are at the level of your belly button (as if holding a beach ball). Bend your legs and push off the ground with your feet, lifting up through the crown of the head, straightening your legs as you jump, and extending through the feet. Try to resist your body from wanting to bend forward by lifting up through the chest. Imagine you are a horse on a carousel and you want to maintain the integrity of your spine while jumping.

This is a great thyroid/metabolism booster.

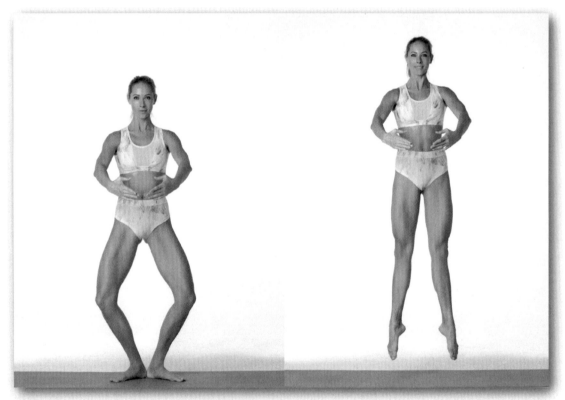

Start with three to five jumps and build up to thirty seconds of consecutive jumps, then repeat three to five times.

KUNDALINI YOGA SQUATS

Start with your feet parallel and as wide as your mat. As you inhale, raise your arms above your head and look up. As you exhale, begin to bend your legs into a deep squat and bring hands to prayer at your chest. If you are unable to get your heels down, then place a folded blanket under your heels. Try to keep your feet parallel and your chest lifted up. At the bottom of the squat, you can press your elbows against your legs to help you lengthen your spine and open up your hips. Then fold forward over yourself, keeping the legs bent, and slowly roll yourself up to stand. Letting your head be the last thing to come up. Repeat three to ten times, depending on how much stuff you need to work through.

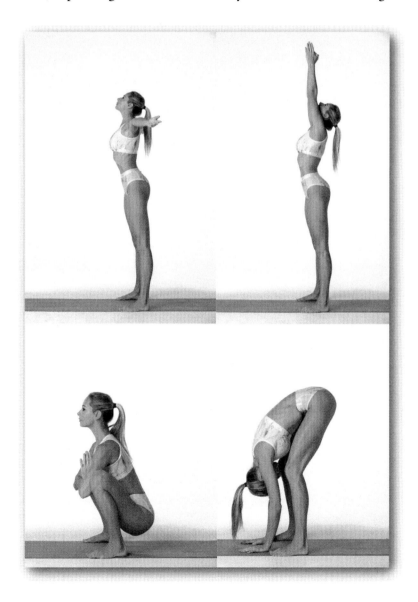

SLOW ROLL SIT-UPS

Start sitting down, with your legs bent, feet flat on the floor and hip-width apart. Bring your arms directly overhead, lengthening evenly on both sides of the body and feeling your sit bones equally on the floor. As you lift your arms up, draw your shoulders away from your ears. Then slowly begin to roll the spine by rounding the back and hollowing the belly, naval to the spine, until you are lying down on the ground with arms overhead. Keep drawing tailbone down and lower ribs in. Just as you came down, begin to roll yourself back up to where you started with your arms overhead. Strive to sit up as tall as you can without any roundness in the spine, before going back down. Continue for one minute.

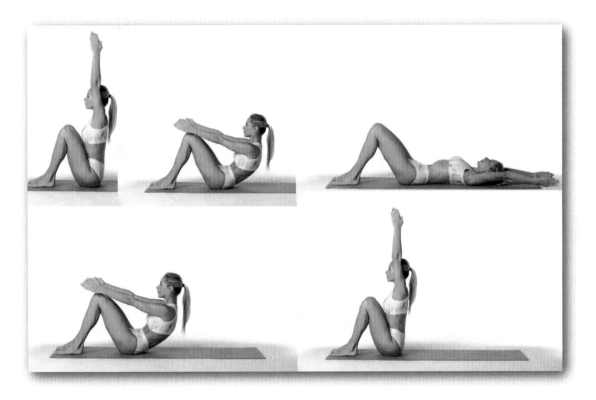

DANDASANA TO CRAB

Start by sitting down with your legs straight out in front of you, knees pointing upward and feet flexed. Arms are alongside your body, directly underneath your shoulders, and palms flat on the ground. Sit up tall by pressing your hands and sit bones into the ground and by lifting up through both sides of your body equally. If this is challenging for you and you are unable to get the roundness out of your lower back, sit on the edge of a folded blanket.

Keeping your hands where they are, begin to lift your hip bones up toward the sky until your feet are flat on the floor. Let your head fall back, if it is comfortable. Press your hands and feet into the ground to help open and lift up the front of your body. Hold for one to two breaths and then return to dandasana. Continue slowly and steady for thirty seconds, building up to one minute.

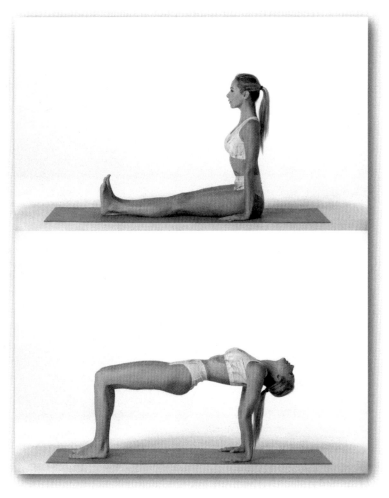

BOAT POSE TO LIFT-UPS (*Navasana*)

Begin by sitting on your bum, legs together and bent. Bring your hands underneath your legs and begin to lean back. Use your arms to help you lift up and get the roundness out of your lower spine. As you lean back, begin to straighten the legs, arms out in front of you. If this is too challenging, then continue to hold onto your legs and focus on finding your balance. Hold three counts then place your hands underneath your shoulders, cross your legs and hug them into your chest. Press the hands into the ground and try to lift up your body by drawing the navel to the spine (as if someone punched you in the stomach). This is very challenging, and at first you may not lift off at all, which is totally normal. A moderation is to use two yoga blocks under your hands to help you press up higher. Also if you have tight legs, hugging them into your chest will be difficult at first so as you gain flexibility this too will become easier. Repeat two more times, coming to boat pose in between press ups.

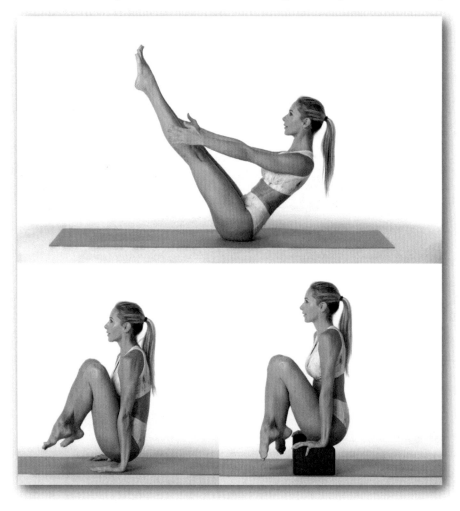

BRIDGE POSE (*Setu Bandha Sarvangasana*)

Start by laying on your back with your feet flat on the floor and toes in, heels out slightly. Press your hips off the floor and bring your arms underneath your back. Clasp your hands together, wiggle the shoulders underneath your chest and straighten the arms back out, pressing them into the ground. With the weight in your heels, lift your hips up to the ceiling, focusing on opening your upper back (heart) then gently press your head into the ground so that your chin is away from your chest. Stay for three to five breaths, then release the clasp of your hands and slowly roll down vertebrae by vertebrae. Bring your feet as wide as your mat then let your knees fall into each other for two breaths before repeating two more times. After the last bridge, bring your legs into your chest and give yourself a big hug, rolling side to side if it feels good.

For the more advanced, you can come into full wheel pose (*urdhva dhanurasana*) by bringing your hands alongside your ears. Press your hands and feet into the ground and pause at the top of your head. Readjust your feet so that your toes point straight forward and hug your elbows toward your ears. Then begin to straighten the arms and legs to come into the full pose. Once you are up, release your inner thighs down and allow your body to open up. Always warm up with at least one bridge pose first.

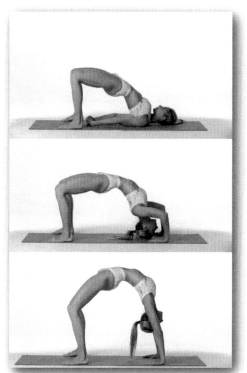

Stretch it out for long and lean muscles with optimal mobility. Age with grace.

THREAD THE NEEDLE

Begin by laying on your back with both feet flat on the floor. Bring your right leg over your left to make a triangle with your legs. Bring your right hand through that triangle and hold onto your left knee with both hands clasped together. Keeping both feet flexed and active to protect your knees, begin to draw your right leg toward your chest. Try to maintain a long spine from your tailbone to the crown of your head. Stay for several breaths, then repeat the same thing on the other side.

This is a great pose to relieve sciatica and any pain associated with the back and outer gluteus maximus and other hip muscles.

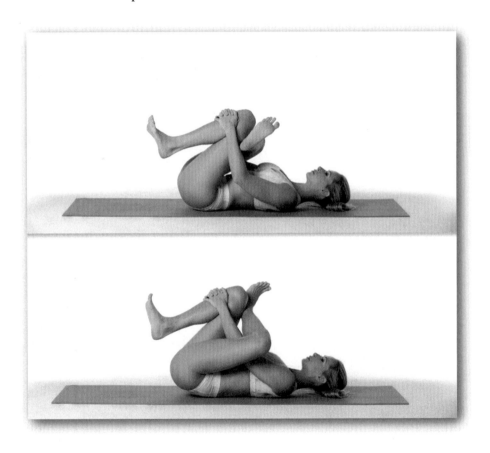

RECLINING HAND-TO-BIG-TOE POSE (*Supta Padangusthasana*)

Use a strap or a long towel. Start by laying on your back with the strap around the outside of your right foot with the ends of the strap in both hands. Bring the right leg straight up to the sky, leaving the left leg on the ground, straight and foot flexed. Begin to draw the right leg toward your chest by bending your elbows out to the sides. Stay a minimum of thirty seconds. Than bring the strap into your right hand and bring your left hand to the top of your left thigh, encouraging it to stay down as you bring your right leg to the side. Stay a minimum of fifteen seconds. Then come back through the center and then bring the strap into your left hand and bring your right leg all the way across your chest to stretch the outside of your leg. Try to get the right arm and shoulder onto the ground and gaze at the right hand. Again holding for a minimum of fifteen seconds. Come back to center and give one last stretch by lifting your chest up and trying to bring your nose to your knee. Repeat on left side. These are minimum times to stay in each stretch, as you build strength and flexibility begin to stay in these stretches for a longer time.

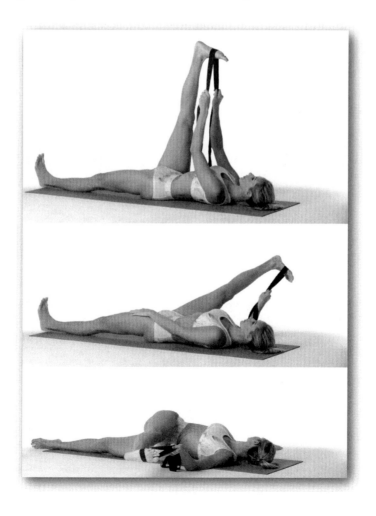

SIMPLE TWISTS LYING DOWN

Start by laying on your back and cross your right leg over your left. Then shift your hips to the right and let your legs fall to the left. Bring your arms straight out to the sides, trying to get the right shoulder onto the ground. Turn your gaze toward your right hand if neck permits. Stay a minimum of thirty seconds, v   repeat on the other side.

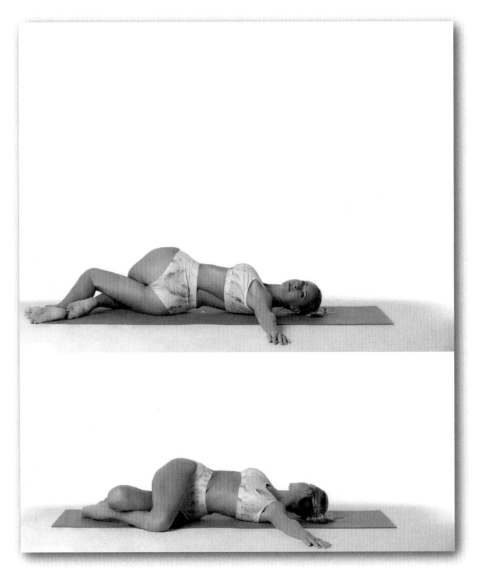

Twisting helps to remove and eliminate built-up toxins from the body. It is not recommended for expecting mothers.

LEGS-UP-THE-WALL POSE (*Viparita Karani*)

You will need a solid wall to do this pose. Start by getting your bum as close to the wall as possible then bring your legs straight up toward the ceiling so that both your bum and legs are flush against the wall. If you tend to get headaches or have tight shoulders and hold tension in your neck, then bring your arms overhead and let them lay on the floor above you. After several breaths you can place your hands onto your belly. Stay as long as you like or until your feet start to tingle. From here you can either bring your legs into your chest and roll to one side to get out of it or for more opening in your hamstrings, let your legs open up to the sides coming into a wide leg split. Stay for a minimum of thirty seconds then when you are ready to get out, place your hands on the outsides of your legs and help them back up the wall. Bring your legs into your chest and give yourself a big hug. Then roll to one side or the other to mindfully get yourself back up to a simple seated position.

This is a passive restorative inversion that helps to reverse the effects of gravity on the entire body, thereby increasing circulation to your heart, abdomen, and lungs as well as helping to balance and stimulate the adrenal glands and kidneys and energizing your entire body—even encouraging blood flow to the face, helping your skin to glow. Great to do after a long day!

Modify: If your hamstrings are tight, then the legs can be on an angle slightly away from the wall.

Variations: Place a bolster, pillow, or folded blanket under your bum to help open the chest up even more.

Yoga teaches us to cure what need not be endured and endure what cannot be cured.

—*B. K. S. Iyengar*

CLOSING MEDITATION

Sit in a comfortable seated position (*sukhasana*). Lengthen your spine from your tailbone to the crown of your head. Place your hands together in prayer with your thumbs pressing against your chest. Close your eyes and notice how different you feel from the start of your practice.

Bring your hands to your forehead, honoring yourself for practicing today and having gratitude that you are able.

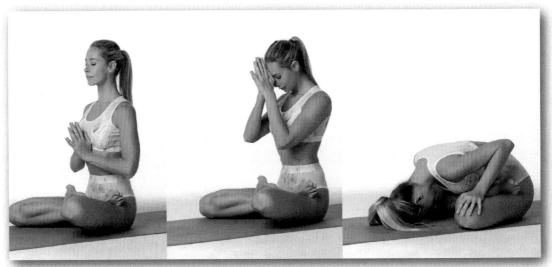

Sequence photos by Todd Vitti

Namaste. *I bow to the divine light within you.*

Part 4
Heal

Let Go

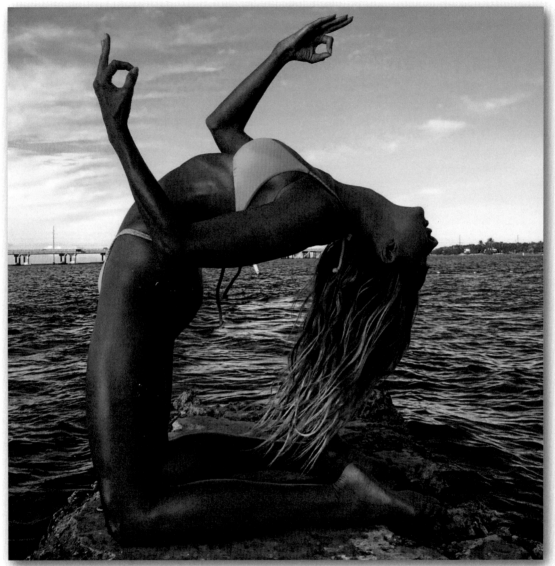

Photo by Maryann Golden

Y ou can only be given the tools, but you must do the work to heal yourself. Let go of the thoughts that make you weak.

I believe that for every ailment and habit we have, they are sourced by some experience we have had or mental pattern (good or bad) that we have created.

The negative emotions and mental patterns that cause the most dis-ease in our body are anger, resentment, self-loathing, and judgment. These feelings can stem from a variety of experiences in our lives. Identifying what those experiences were, or are, are crucial in order to prevent, heal, and get rid of addictive behaviors and other behaviors that do not serve us.

Often these experiences are ones that we would rather forget, but in order to dissolve the mental cause, we need to look inside and remove it from its roots. Our instincts usually know the connections right away, but in order to detour the pain that may arise during the healing process, we put a bandage on the problem and carry on until the symptoms get bigger. I believe not "removing the roots" of the problem is often the reason why medicine, sugar, and recovery programs don't work. We are just cutting the weeds (covering up the symptoms) and not going deep enough to get to the core or root of the problem.

This takes more than discipline and willpower. It takes a willingness to release and let go of anything negative in our lives. It takes courage to allow yourself to feel emotions that you have been avoiding, and it takes practice to retrain your brain and break old patterns.

Our thoughts are very powerful. What we think in the present moment becomes our future. This awareness is what we may need to motivate us to develop and create new, healthy thought patterns and experiences.

Positive affirmations are very useful. We can't just will the thoughts and habits away; we must replace them with positive ones.

Louise Hay has written about how our thoughts relate to metaphysical causes for different body ailments. Her book *You Can Heal Your Life* is a must-read. In this book Louise not only describes the connection between thoughts and bodily issues, but she provides positive affirmations to help dissolve the mental patterns that caused the ailment.

The practice of daily affirmations changes our thinking patterns, thereby changing our experience. Perhaps, at first, you may feel awkward saying positive affirmations, but that may be an indication that you could really benefit from them. Even if you don't believe what you are saying at first, keep saying it until you do believe it.

Studies say it takes twenty-one days to break a habit.

Give positive affirmations a chance for twenty-one days and see how you feel at the end of the twenty-one days! *Letting go is the hardest asana.*

REFLECT

Do you have any ailments?

_____

List each one of them.

_____

_____

_____

_____

What emotional experience in your life do you think is associated to each ailment listed? Go with your first instinct. Don't question yourself.

_____

_____

_____

_____

Now, replace each negative emotion and agreement you made with yourself with a new, positive, healthy one. Most often the cure is the opposite emotion of what you originally believed.

_____

_____

_____

_____

Get Some Sunlight

I believe in the sun! The sun is a powerful healing resource. Ever since I was a child, I relied on the sun to help me feel good and energized. Unfortunately the sun gets a bum rap because of its association with the risk of skin cancer and premature signs of aging.

Sunlight is an essential element that we need in order to survive. Sunlight is very healing, disinfecting, and energizing. The healing power of the sun is capable of killing many kinds of bacteria and giving you an overall feeling of wellness.

We also get the important nutrient vitamin D from the sun. Despite its name, vitamin D is actually a steroid hormone precursor. The recommended amount of sunlight, to get an adequate amount of vitamin D, is twenty minutes per day. This twenty-minute exposure is without chemically filled sunscreens blocking the sun's assimilation. In just twenty minutes your body is able to receive the sun's health benefits, which include increased bone health and immune function and, contrary to popular belief, decreased risk of cancer. Vitamin D deficiency has been linked to many autoimmune disorders, such as lupus, rheumatoid arthritis, and multiple sclerosis.

If you live in a Northern climate or are exposed to minimal sunlight, then you may require additional vitamin D. In fact, most of us are deficient in vitamin D no matter how much sunlight we get. This may be due to the fact that our body does not assimilate vitamin D properly. This is where vitamin K2 comes in. Vitamin K2 helps to get vitamin D to the place it needs to get…to your bones.

Natural sources of vitamin K2 include fermented veggies and organic *natto* (fermented soybean).

Exposure to sunlight encourages every important function of the body to work at its best. When we absorb the sun's rays into our skin, it stores up energy in our body. Our nerves absorb the energy and transmit it to our entire body.

Lack of sunshine can also make you SAD, literally! Lack of natural sunlight can cause a nervous, melancholy disorder called SAD (seasonal affective disorder). People who are not exposed to natural sunlight due to either their desire to stay indoors or where they live could develop SAD. SAD can progress into full-blown panic disorders and/or depression.

Research shows that people who live or work in a place where they are exposed to lots of natural light are less depressed, healthier, and more productive.

HOW TO MAXIMIZE YOUR SUN EXPOSURE:

- Be mindful not to overexpose your skin to the sun. Start with five minutes a day and build up to twenty minutes. You never want to get burned.

- Choose toxin-free, mineral-based sunscreens, available at most health food stores. Most mainstream sunscreens contain oxybenzone, a chemical that can disrupt your hormones and cause allergies, skin irritations, and low birth weight in newborn girls.

- Choose natural oils that act as a sunscreen, such as:

  - Carrot seed oil, SPF 40

  - Red raspberry oil, SPF between 30 and 50

  - Avocado oil, SPF 4–10

  - Coconut oil, SPF 2–8

  - Olive oil, SPF 2–8

  - Almond oil, SPF 5

The sun will continue to rise and set. What we choose to do with the sunlight is up to us.

REFLECT

How to slowly make each day better.

1. Make a list of the things that make you happy.

_____

_____

_____

_____

_____

2. Make a list of the things you do every day.

_____

_____

_____

_____

3. Compare the lists and adjust accordingly.

_____

_____

_____

_____

Nature First

I'm not suggesting you throw out all your over-the-counter drugs, but I am suggesting that you leave them as a last resort. I am saying use natural remedies for chronic or common ailments, not emergency scenarios when Western medicine is needed. *Always seek professional medical help in an emergency.*

Nurture with nature. I believe nature cures when a cure is possible.

For minor ailments, try natural remedies first, and only if that fails turn to over-the-counter or pharmaceutical drugs.

Many pharmaceutical drugs mask or cover up problems, often creating more health issues in the long run. Pharmaceuticals often also have significant side effects. When you have side effects, you are treating the side effects in addition to your original ailment, creating a cycle of dependency on drugs that may have a harsh effect on your body. I do believe there is a place for some pharmaceutical drugs, but I believe they are highly overused and should be used as a last resort, not as a first resort.

Holistic remedies help the body naturally fight infections, building up one's natural immunity. I recommend treating a person holistically, healing and extending one's life through nature's cures.

THE GOLDEN SECRETS NATURAL FIRST AID KIT FOR THE HOME

COLLOIDAL SILVER
A natural antibiotic and my first resource for cuts, scrapes, and the first sign of any illness. I even use it as a facial mist during acne breakouts. Colloidal silver is known for naturally killing bacteria.

Reserve antibiotics for acute bacterial infections. Overuse of antibiotics promotes the development of drug-resistant bacteria.

CAYENNE TINCTURE
My "go to" for breaking up congestion, opening up the blood flow, and reducing bleeding. Cayenne provides an excellent source of vitamin C and can be added to your morning juicing. Cayenne can even improve brain function.

Cayenne and other spices with zest can clear sinuses, improve circulation and blood flow, and give your metabolism a kick.

GARLIC
A staple in the Mediterranean diet, garlic has many health benefits, from aiding the immune system to helping with various cancers and heart disease. Garlic can kill almost anything! Eat it fresh and eat it often.

Folklore prescribes using garlic and olive oil on a sick person's feet to reduce a fever. After rubbing the concoction on the ill person's feet, one would place socks or wrap towels on the feet to hold the ingredients in place. It was believed that the garlic would pull the illness out of the body by using the feet as an easy exit point.

ONIONS
Not an apple a day, but an onion a day. Onions have antibiotic and antiseptic properties; they lower cholesterol, can relieve respiratory problems, and alleviate pain and inflammation. In addition to being internally effective, an onion is so potent that it is known to absorb toxins from the air.

At the first sign of a cold, cut an onion in half, placing half of it near your bed while you sleep. Change the onion every three days if you are using it for multiple days.

APPLE CIDER VINEGAR
Use raw, organic, unfiltered, and unpasteurized apple cider vinegar for many health, beauty, and household benefits. Made from fermented apples, this vinegar can help balance and maintain a healthy alkaline pH level in your body, giving you more energy, helping your body rid itself of toxins, and aiding in optimal weight management.

Try these other uses for apple cider vinegar: as a room freshener, a flea repellant, to reduce heartburn, to help rid the body of candida, to help break up mucus, as a natural anti-inflammatory, or to help eliminate sunburn discomfort. Apply externally for glowing skin and hair.

Rinse your mouth after drinking apple cider vinegar as it can break down your teeth enamel.

ASTRAGALUS ROOT

Used in traditional Chinese medicine for the common cold, viral infections, chronic diarrhea, diabetes, and to help lower blood pressure. Cancer patients using traditional Western treatment sometimes use astragalus root to help restore immune function. It is an overall immune booster and often made into a tonic to act as a white blood cell builder.

Chinese medicine, such as Chinese herbal formulas and acupuncture, can help balance the immune system by rebalancing the flow of *qi* (life force).

OREGANO OIL

Known to have powerful antioxidant and anticancer properties, oregano oil can also be used externally in baths to relieve aches and pains associated with stiff joints. Studies show that it is as effective as antibiotics in the treatment of certain bacterial infections.

Immunity shots with oregano oil have been proven to help fight common colds and infections. Oregano oil has quite a kick and can give your mouth and lips a tingle.

MEDICINAL MUSHROOMS

Asian mushrooms such as reishi, shiitake, and maitake and cordyceps all have anti-inflammatory, antiviral, and anticancer properties. I recommend cooking all mushrooms prior to eating them to remove toxins and to make them more digestible.

Dried mushrooms can be reconstituted in water and sautéed or baked. Mushroom extracts can be added to broths and teas.

LYSINE

An amino acid that inhibits the growth of the herpes virus, as well as Epstein-Barr infections (another virus in the herpes family). Lysine is needed for proper tissue repair and enzyme production and is found naturally in brewers' yeast and milk products. It can be used for maintenance, but also for the occasional virus when strong immune support is needed.

Lysine inhibits the growth of herpes, whereas arginine encourages it. Steer clear of food with arginine when the immune system is compromised. Some foods containing arginine are chocolate, peanuts, most nuts and even some grains.

ECHINACEA
Known for fighting infections, especially the common cold. Echinacea can also be helpful with chronic fatigue syndrome, migraines, yeast infections, and the flu.

ZINC
Known for fighting common colds. Zinc can also be helpful with reoccurring ear infections, eczema, acne, ADHD (attention deficit/hyperactivity disorder), and diabetes.

Excessive doses of zinc can suppress the immune system and cause digestive disturbance, so be sure to take the proper amount for your body.

RAW ORGANIC HONEY
Unprocessed honey contains pollen, propolis, and live enzymes. If you suffer from allergies and are able to get local honey, it could be your antidote. Raw honey is also great for the immune system and especially soothing to sore throats.

LEMON
An alkaline food with numerous health benefits and loaded with vitamin C. Drinking warm water with lemon in the morning can help cleanse your intestinal tract. Use lemon during a cold or flu. Lemon is especially good for reducing coughing. There is nothing better for a constant cough than raw honey and lemon juice, unless codeine is prescribed.

Lemon juice can erode teeth enamel so don't hold it in your mouth for a prolonged amount of time and be sure to rinse your mouth out after you are finished drinking the juice.

GINGER
Known to help with cancer, migraines, and nausea, ginger is a strong anti-inflammatory and also helpful for the common cold and flu. When bathing with ginger or drinking it in hot tea, ginger increases perspiration, which helps to remove toxins from the body.

FENNEL
Have you ever heard of gripe water? It is used to cure colic in babies. Gripe water is made from brewed fennel seeds and is effective for babies as well as adults. Digestive and gastrointestinal upsets, flatulence, bloating, and menstrual disorders can be naturally relieved by fennel. Also used as an appetite-suppressant, it can be effective for those who are overweight.

NETI POT
Nasal cleansing with warm water and sea salt in a neti pot can be used when congestion and difficulty breathing is prominent, or for sinus infections. It is also used as a purifier to clear nasal passages from pollution, dust, and pollen. The neti pot is also used to prevent allergies, asthma, and other respiratory problems.

ESSENTIAL OILS
The essence or essential oil of a plant is said to capture the very life force of the plant itself. So when you use essential oils, your body, mind, and emotions attune to the very energy of the plant. Each plant offers a wide range of properties, or effects, yet each of us draws from these properties individually, depending on our own needs, harmonizing to your particular constitution and amplifying the potential to heal. Completely shifting your mind-body dynamic in a positive way and raising your electromagnetic frequency.

SOME COMMON ESSENTIAL OILS ARE THE FOLLOWING:

- Lavender oil, which is beneficial in helping one to relax and sleep, can reduce a cold, digestive problems, and earaches.

- Lemon oil can energize and help sharpen your memory, fight inflammation, and is also great for respiratory issues.

- Rosemary and eucalyptus oils can reduce mucus production and heal other respiratory issues like asthma.

- Ylang-ylang oil has been shown to stimulate the release of feel-good endorphins.

- Grapefruit oil has been shown to increase your threshold for pain and ease motion sickness.

- Peppermint oil is great for reducing fevers, preventing a cold, and relieving sinus congestion or infection.

Always dilute essential oils before applying to the skin. Mix with a carrier oil and massage onto the area in question, or add to a diffuser.

HOMEOPATHIC REMEDIES
Homeopathy is based on the principle that "like cures like," called the Law of Contraries. The Law of Contraries proposes that an illness should be treated by a substance capable of

producing similar symptoms to what the sick person is suffering from. Homeopathy does not cover up the symptoms of an illness, but rather works by helping the body's defense system to help itself. It is a safe, natural way to treat the whole body with no negative side effects. If you choose the wrong remedy, it will simply not work.

Arnica montana is one of the most common remedies used for bruises, sprains, and strains. There are 105 homeopathic remedies, but some are not widely available. There are thirty common remedies for minor, everyday complaints and fifteen key remedies used for a wide range of general ailments and long-term conditions.

FLOWER REMEDIES
Dr. Edward Bach has discovered thirty-eight flower remedies designed for particular personality characteristics or for one's emotional state. Flower remedies are a great resource to have on hand for many conditions like stress, grief, lack of confidence, shock, and feeling overwhelmed. Flower remedies are all natural and safe. Just like homeopathic remedies, if it isn't the right remedy, it simply won't work.

Rescue Remedy may be the most common flower remedy on the market and great to have on hand for stress relief.

Color Therapy

The colors that we wear, the colors of the rooms we spend time in, and the colors of the foods we eat have a profound effect on our overall well-being. The colors we see every day can either stimulate or depress the cells in our bodies. It is not a coincidence that certain colors are used for signals, signs, and even uniforms. Doctor scrubs are often blue, as blue is very calming and some of its properties are antiseptic and astringent.

Color therapy consists of all the colors of the rainbow, and each color carries its own frequency or vibration. Colors are able to affect moods, organs, and body parts. Colors also coincide with the seven chakras. These chakras are subtle life force centers within the human energy system.

RED
Enhances physical strength, courage, power, and sexuality. It is energizing and stimulating. Red can be healing because it can increase circulation, raise one's body temperature, correct sexual dysfunctions, and increase hemoglobin (the molecules in red blood cells responsible for transporting oxygen). Associated with the first energy center chakra and located at the root or base of the tailbone.

ORANGE
The color of wisdom that stimulates energy, brings joy, and relieves depression. Can alleviate gastrointestinal problems and help poor assimilation of food. Can be healing for asthma, bronchial issues (coughs), gout, inflammation of joints, and rheumatic aches. Associated with the second energy center chakra and located in the pelvic region or spleen.

YELLOW
Enhances wisdom, knowledge, intelligence, inspiration, health, and patience. Can help heal constipation, diarrhea, liver and pancreas issues. Can also help alleviate eczema and other skin conditions, along with providing adrenal support. The empowering third energy chakra is located at the solar plexus.

GREEN
One of the most healing of all the colors. Green is especially helpful with stimulating the thymus gland, normalizing blood pressure, and assisting with fatigue, influenza, cardiac conditions, ulcers, and controlling one's temper. Helps to stimulate compassion and forgiveness. Represents growth and new beginnings. The fourth chakra is located at the heart and is also associated with the color pink.

BLUE
Represents youth and inspires confidence. Blue is a cold color and is great for healing fevers and high blood pressure. Blue is also healing for headaches, vomiting, insomnia, and throat issues. Blue can help you speak your truth. Blue is the fifth chakra and is located at the throat.

INDIGO
Stimulates the "king" of all the glands, the pineal gland, located in the middle of the eyebrows and is sometimes called the "third eye." This sixth energy chakra is also associated with the colors purple and violet. This sixth chakra stimulates one's intuition, insight, spirituality, adventure, and prosperity. It also influences the eyes, ears, and nose. Indigo is an astringent, a cooling and purifying color, that helps broaden one's mind, free inhibitions, and alleviate serious obsessions.

VIOLET
Believed to be the highest vibrational color and is found at the crown of the head. This seventh chakra color is associated with understanding and bliss. Violet is linked to the pituitary gland, intuition, and spirituality. This chakra color is healing for mental and nervous disorders, like concussions and neurosis. The crown chakra is also associated with the colors gold and white.

WHITE
Represents purity, innocence, and new beginnings. White is cleansing and makes one feel whole, free, and light. The seventh chakra disperses energy to the lower six chakras, bringing mindfulness, consciousness, and creation to what the mind can conceive. White consists of the entire spectrum of colors.

BLACK
Black is a contemplative color that encourages introspection and reflection. Representing the void, it is protective, mysterious, and secretive. Keeping you hidden, it is not a color to wear when you want to express yourself and feel uplifted.

BROWN

Represents the Earth. Brown is nurturing, grounding, and rooted. Brown is great for a wandering mind and inability to focus. As an earth tone, it is not a color to wear when you want to expand or branch out.

Colors, like features, follow the changes of the emotions.—Pablo Picasso

REFLECT

What colors do you wear most often?

_____

_____

_____

_____

_____

_____

What colors are you going to start wearing and surrounding yourself with?

_____

_____

_____

_____

_____

_____

Clear Negative Energy

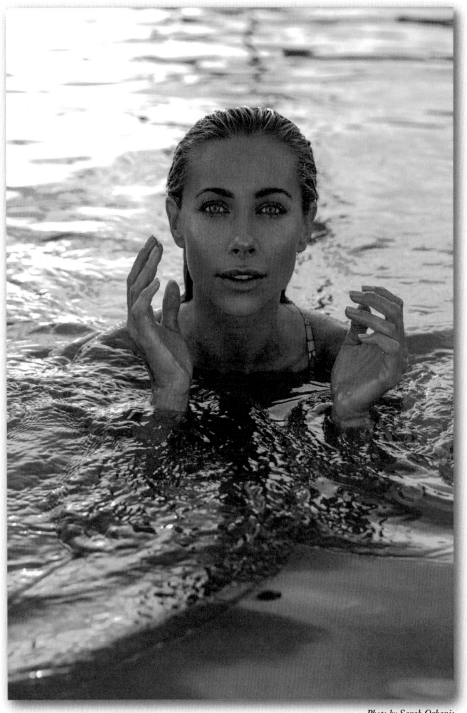

Photo by Sarah Orbanic

We are subconsciously picking up other people's energies all the time. Have you ever walked into a room and felt negative energy? Or had an argument with someone and felt the tension in the air? Without knowing how to properly protect, transmute, and remove these negative energies, they could affect your overall health and state of mind.

HERE ARE SOME WAYS TO PREVENT AND RELEASE NEGATIVE ENERGY YOU MAY BE CARRYING:

SMUDGING
Burning incense, sage, mugwort, or sandalwood sticks is found in many traditions but is mostly known from North American native traditions, specifically those that include shamanism. They are used in ceremonial rituals to clear negative spirits and energy.

- With sage or an herb of your choice in hand, light a small piece of it and blow out, always keeping a tray or abalone shell underneath it to catch any ash.

- Walk around your house, or the area you wish to cleanse, and let the smoke get to every corner.

- Most importantly, sage yourself and be sure to sage under your feet. Always leave a window or door open so that the smoke has a place to exit.

During the Renaissance, courtesans would use burning sage, standing over the smoke in their long dresses, to clear their "hoo-hah" between pleasuring men. They believed that the smoking sage would protect them from any sickness.

BELLS
The ringing of bells is a common feng shui tool known to vibrate negative energies into alignment and create a positive flow. Ring a bell throughout your house or in a specific area where a negative situation occurred.

Raising your glasses and "clinking" them originated in the Middle Ages when people believed that alcoholic drinks contained spirits. The "clinking" of the glasses was thought to rid the alcohol of any spirits, making them safe to drink.

SALT WATER BATHS
Have you ever noticed how happy surfers or people living by the ocean appear to be? Maybe it's because they are continually being cleared by the ocean water. If you don't have access to the ocean, add salt to a bath.

- Soak in a warm tub with a handful of unprocessed sea salt, Epsom salt, or Dead Sea minerals. Do not use table salt!

- Set an intention to release all negativity while you are soaking. Visualize your aura (the energy surrounding your physical body) being cleansed until the water gets cool. Then imagine all that negative energy going down the drain with the water.

- After soaking, notice how much lighter and clearer you feel. Dry off thoroughly and put a robe on right after your bath to seal in the heat and ATTAIN THE MOST BENEFITS.

CRYSTALS

Crystals have been used for thousands of years to heal, strengthen, and help dispel, absorb, and remove negative energy. You can wear them as jewelry for healing and assisting with clarity. Keep one in your pocket or purse for grounding, or place them in areas of your home that you want to be ignited with positive energy. They are superchargers and help release trapped negative energy, achieving harmony and flow. There are many varieties of crystals and each possesses its own unique vibration, color, shape, and healing energy.

When you get a new crystal, it is important that you smudge it, put it in the sun, or place it in salt water to cleanse it (though some crystals can disintegrate in salt water so be mindful not to submerge it for too long). This will release any energy from the previous owner.

CUTTING CORDS

We all have invisible energetic attachments to those in our lives, and they are called "cords." Some of these cords are beautiful, light, and feed you positive energy; some feed you negative energy, and it is these negative cords that could cause harm.

We develop these cords with everyone we know and have ever known. Have you ever noticed that as soon as you start to date again after a breakup, the ex-boyfriend suddenly calls or texts you? When that happens to me, I believe he must have felt it when I was "cutting his cord" and moving on. Whether we are aware of it or not, we carry these cords from past relationships, unless we detach from them.

With negative cords, visualizing them retracting back to you is one way to get your power back, but visualizing cutting the cord with a pair of scissors can do the trick too. It may seem silly at first, but with real or imaginary scissors, cut the cords that may have negative attachments. By literally making the physical motion of cutting the cords, you start the process of releasing these negative energies that your subconscious is holding onto.

I visualize these cords coming from my solar plexus (third chakra), but there are no rules, so go with your own instinct as to where these cords are stemming from and detach the cords from there.

PROTECT YOURSELF

Surround your entire body with a white bubble. Allow it to extend out to your loved ones, your country, and the planet. Your positive thoughts and intentions matter and send protection out into the world.

Another protection tool is to imagine that there are mirrors facing outward all around you so that any negativity is reflected back to where it came from, thus not allowing that negativity to be absorbed by you. It is like the grade school slogan, *whatever you say to me, bounces off of me and sticks to you like glue.* I especially love this tool for kids in order to teach them to protect themselves from negative energy.

I always tell my son, "The bugs are attracted to the light. You are the light and you need to protect yourself."

High Frequency Sounds

All matter has a unique vibration and is in constant motion. Everything moves, vibrates and circles. This motion generates frequencies, which then generates sound, even if we don't hear it. Every chakra has a sound that tunes to that particular part of the body. The first sounds we hear in the womb sounds similar to static radio noise (white noise). That is why a static radio can instantly calm a crying baby.

Studies show that although humans cannot hear ultrasound (sounds at frequencies above approximately twenty kilohertz,) ultrasound can play a large role in a person's overall health. The human body has an electrical frequency and a person's health is determined by that frequency.

Cancer research discovered that human cells have an electric voltage.

The average frequency of a healthy body ranges from sixty-two to seventy-eight megahertz. A person suffering from an illness or disease will have a much lower frequency, starting at fifty-eight megahertz.

Studies have shown that eating unhealthy foods and having negative thoughts can lower your frequency as much as twelve megahertz, while healthy food choices and positive thoughts can raise one's frequency as much as ten megahertz. High frequency sounds may have the capability to heal and repair your DNA by releasing toxins and cleansing your body.

We use music to make us feel different emotions. It can make us cry, give us chills, or psyche us up for a workout. These feelings release beneficial neuropeptides from our brain and these neuropeptides enhance our immune function.

Honored by the ancients, frequency medicine is a powerful sound healing modality that has the potential to bring you to an expanded state of consciousness. Bringing forth insight and relief from physical and emotional pain. The benefits of this heightened state can remain for days after the initial exposure.

BRAINWAVE FREQUENCIES

We all have five different brain wave frequencies: beta, alpha, theta, delta, and gamma. Each frequency is measured in cycles per second (hertz) and each has a unique and specific level of brain consciousness. Learning about the deeper states of consciousness allows us to create the reality we desire.

BETA (14-40 hertz)

The waking state when we are aware of time and space and all of our five senses. We are active in a conversation or engaging our mental and verbal skills.

Beta is the state that most adults operate in. In this state we can do complex problem solving and other tasks that demand our full attention.

Small children and animals function primarily in the alpha, theta, and delta states of mind.

ALPHA (7.5-14 hertz)

Time and space becomes unlimited, as in nap time, light sleep, and meditation. It is when we are tapped into our inner wisdom. The voice of alpha is our intuition.

The alpha state often becomes a pattern after complex thinking or experiencing stress or when an intention has been made to focus on oneself, away from outside influences. This state naturally occurs just after waking up and just before falling sleep.

THETA (4-7.5 hertz)

Insight and creative ideas are often realized here, as well as psychic abilities and deeper wisdom. The theta state occurs in deep sleep and meditation.

Children under the age of thirteen are most commonly in this "zoning out" or "daydreaming" theta pattern.

DELTA (0.5-4 hertz)

Occurs in unconscious deep sleep, or deep meditation (transcendental), allowing the body to completely reset, repair, and heal itself.

Most people enter a delta brain pattern after ninety minutes of sleep. The delta state is a deep dreamless sleep.

GAMMA (above 40 hertz)
High level of cognitive function. In this gamma state, intelligence, compassion, self-control, optimism, and a natural state of happiness are attained, as well as peak athletic performance.

Studies show that people suffering from mental challenges and learning disabilities tend to have lower gamma activity.

HOW TO HEAL WITH HIGH FREQUENCY SOUNDS:

SOUND HEALING
Listen to 528 hertz (the love frequency) or 432 hertz (the earth frequency). You can listen to these frequencies while you meditate or sleep, or as background sound at home or work. I use this practice as a tune-up for my soul.

I do not recommend listening to these frequencies while driving a car or doing anything else that requires your full attention.

CHANTING MANTRAS
Charge your human battery and open the door to subconscious healing on a vibrational, cellular level by reciting, playing, or listening to beautiful mantras. Chanting mantras shifts your energy and aids in healing your body, mind, and heart. One of my favorite mantras is *Ong namo guru dev namo*, which means "I bow to the subtle divine wisdom; I bow to the divine teacher within."

GONG THERAPY
The gong is one of the oldest therapeutic instruments. Gong therapy is known to reduce stress, stimulate the glandular system, and facilitate in breaking through emotional blockages. The goal of gong therapy (as it is for many other sound therapies) is to raise our vibrational frequencies, thereby restoring our natural state of balance.

SINGING BOWL
Traditionally used in Buddhist practices, signaling the beginning or the end of silent meditation. Singing bowls clear the energy in a room, allowing for new energy to come in. Singing bowls aid in meditation, yoga, and sound healing.

If you could eliminate outside frequencies that interfered with our bodies, we would have greater resistance toward disease.

—Nikola Tesla

Metal and Gem Therapy

Who would have thought that even the jewelry we wear could affect our health? Metals and gems affect the body's electromagnetic field either positively or negatively. Gold, silver, and copper jewelry energizes the body because of its electron structure and purity. These metals give a person physical strength, as well as stamina and energy.

If you wear bracelets and anklets, wear them on your left side because the natural flow of the electromagnetic field enters the left and leaves the right.

Each gem carries its own energy and healing benefits. This is good to remember, especially when choosing to wear previously owned gems, as the stone can carry the energy (good or bad) of the previous owner. Be aware of how you feel when you wear these gems. Retest your response to these gems every couple of months, either with muscle testing (also known as applied kinesiology, a noninvasive way of evaluating the body's needs) or your intuition, and if needed, smudge or place the gem in the sunlight to cleanse.

Metals such as lead, iron, pewter, and tin should never be worn as jewelry because they tend to shorten one's electromagnetic field causing the person to feel weak and tired. Wearing these metals could eventually cause illness.

Diamonds are known for their beauty and prestige, but they can also strengthen the thymus area or thyroid.

These health benefits add a new perspective to "diamonds are a girl's best friend."

Legend says that wearing a gemstone during its assigned month can heighten its healing and therapeutic powers and can be very complimentary for the wearer.

BELOW ARE THE BIRTHSTONES FOR EACH MONTH:

January	*Garnet*
February	*Amethyst*
March	*Aquamarine*
April	*Diamond*
May	*Emerald*
June	*Pearl/Alexandrite*
July	*Ruby*
August	*Peridot*
September	*Sapphire*
October	*Opal/Tourmaline*
November	*Topaz/Citrine*
December	*Turquoise/Zircon/Tanzanite*

BELOW ARE DESCRIPTIONS OF THE HEALTH BENEFITS FOR SOME OF THE HIGH VIBRATIONAL GEMS:

COPPER
Good for rheumatism, arthritis, gout, and circulation. Copper promotes generosity and is very helpful in removing energy blocks within the body.

GOLD
Great for the heart, cleanses the blood, aids in asthma, reduces sadness, and attracts physical and spiritual energy. *Gold has one of the highest vibrational frequencies and it symbolizes the sun.*

SILVER
Metal of the moon, head, and brain. Silver is good for epilepsy and rheumatism. Silver benefits many, but it does not carry as high a vibration as gold or platinum.

AMETHYST
Helps preserve sobriety and counters negativity. Amethyst is a high vibrational energy stone used by many spiritually minded people due to its help in meditating. Amethyst can increase courage, decrease insomnia, and relieve pain and circulatory issues. Folklore says sleeping with an amethyst next to your bed ensures sweet dreams.

CITRINE
Can create joy and cheerfulness by lifting one's mood. Citrine helps with hearing loss or selective hearing and promotes clear thinking, abundance, and success.

DIAMOND
Can strengthen friendship and love, brings forward courage and strength and can help with degenerative diseases.

OPAL
Clarifies the mind and helps with memory and eyesight. Opal is a high vibrational stone that attracts good fortune in travel and business.

TURQUOISE
Can help relieve tension and provides protection, especially from injury. Turquoise is a high vibrational earth stone that radiates peace and brings balance and self-confidence to the wearer.

> *If you want to find the secrets of the universe, think in terms of energy, frequency, and vibration.*
>
> —NIKOLA TESLA

REFLECT

What is your birthstone?

_____

_____

_____

_____

What jewelry do you wear most often and where do you wear it?

_____

_____

_____

_____

What gems do you think you need to wear more often and where?

_____

_____

_____

_____

Part 5
Mind

Don't Worry

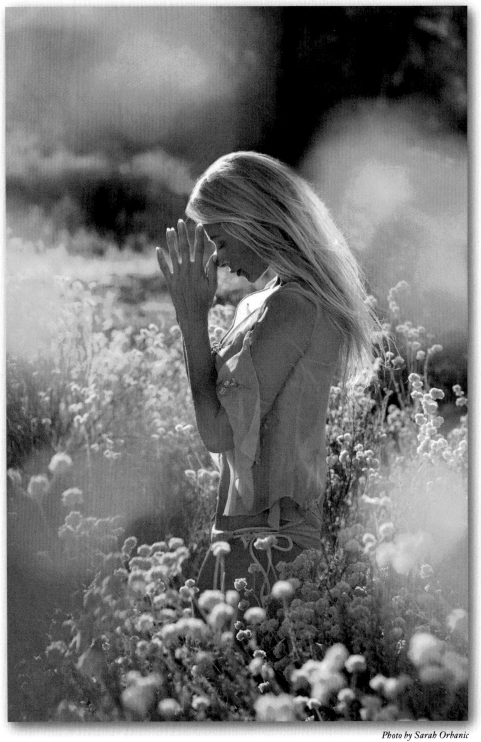

Photo by Sarah Orbanic

The soul usually knows what to do to heal itself. The challenge is to silence the mind.

One of the common denominators in people who live long, healthy, happy lives is their ability to let things roll off their backs.

Worrying does not change a circumstance; it only causes stress. Worrying puts extreme stress on the body. Our bodies may go into "fight or flight" mode, releasing cortisone, and over time this response can cause numerous health issues. There will always be something to worry about if you choose to let yourself go there. People who do not worry, don't necessarily have less to worry about, they just choose to perceive things differently. They surrender to the universe and have faith in a higher power.

Worrying and not worrying are learned habits. In order to change your behavior, you must retrain your brain's triggers.

EVERY TIME YOU FIND YOURSELF WORRYING, TRY ONE OF THESE TACTICS:

- Find comfort in a higher power.

- Repeat a mantra or a positive affirmation.

- Remind yourself that the last time you spent time worrying, everything ended up working out.

- Visualize a positive outcome. Imagine every detail as you desire it to be. The more detailed your picture the better: include colors, scents, smells, flavors, textures, feelings, and emotions. Practice visualizing often, especially when a negative thought comes in.

- Be mindful of your thoughts and reroute your mind back to your desired outcome. Issues will always arise, but you can change your reaction to them. Have gratitude for the positive things you do have and focus on those. Only give water to the seeds you want to grow.

- Practice tuning in (meditation) every day. Start with five minutes and build up to twenty minutes. Simplify your meditation by just sitting still and letting your thoughts come and go. Steady breath, steady mind. Notice if your breath is shallow. Focus on your breath until your worries dissipate. Try breathing in a 4-7-8 pattern:

- Inhale for four seconds.

- Hold the breath for seven seconds.

- Exhale for eight seconds.

- Practice yoga, walking, or some kind of physical exercise to help you release your stress in a constructive way.

- Use essential oils such as lavender, chamomile, valerian, bergamot, clary sage, frankincense, nutmeg, neroli, rose, and jasmine. Through their scent, essential oils have a profound healing, nourishing, and comforting effect. Add several drops of your favorite to a warm bath. Add several drops to a carrier oil, such as almond oil, and apply to your feet and hands. Add to a vaporizer or place several drops onto a handkerchief and inhale throughout the day.

- Try natural, holistic remedies like Rescue Remedy or other flower essences that treat your specific issues. Also investigate supplementing the nutrients calcium, magnesium, potassium, selenium, B-complex vitamins, vitamins C and E, and zinc into your diet to help calm and de-stress you.

- Drink herbal teas with ashwagandha, valerian root, passionflower, holy basil, or other stress-relieving adaptogens. Steer clear of excess caffeine or stimulating products as they can cause nervous tension and unwanted anxiety, a breeding ground for worry.

The secret of health for both mind and body is not to mourn for the past, worry about the future, or anticipate troubles, but to live in the present moment wisely and earnestly.

—*PARAMAHANSA YOGANANDA*

REFLECT

List three things you always find yourself worrying about.

_____

_____

_____

_____

Now write your ideal outcome for each.

_____

_____

_____

_____

_____

_____

_____

_____

Every time you find yourself retreating back to a worried thought, replace that thought with your desired outcome.

Laugh

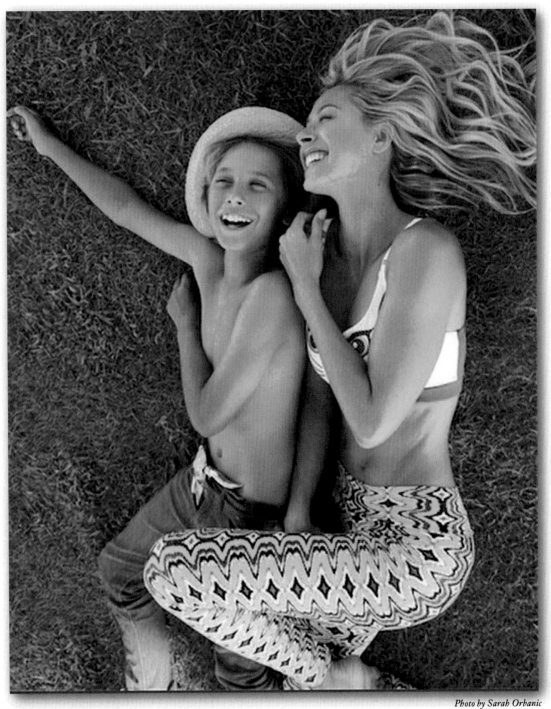

Photo by Sarah Orbanic

Laugh your bum off. Literally! Laughing burns fifty calories in ten to fifteen minutes. Laughing has anti-stress capabilities by easing the body's stress response and preserving immune function. Studies show that even if you "fake laugh," you receive the benefits. Some of the oldest people in the world say that finding joy in the simple, everyday things in life and *laughing* is what keeps them young and healthy.

- Watch a funny movie, have a game night, or go to a comedy show.

- Surround yourself with people who you can be goofy with and who make you laugh.

- Have a laughing party! Yes, it's a thing. Invite your friends over and have everybody lay on the ground in a circle. Then have each person lay his or her head on the next person's belly. Start laughing and in no time the whole group will be uncontrollably laughing.

- Better yet, film the laughing party and then laugh all over again while you crack up watching you and your friends crack up.

- Spend time with children and let yourself be immersed in their silliness. Children remind us to be carefree and encourage us to be goofy. They find the simplest things funny. A simple game of peekaboo can be the most hilarious thing in the world to young children.

- Participate in fun activities, like karaoke or bowling, or go to an amusement park and experience a ride that you wouldn't normally go on.

- Don't take yourself or life too seriously. Enjoy your life and allow yourself to laugh along the way!

- Smile in adversity. That is one of my secrets to staying uplifted.

The ultimate goal is to laugh as much as you breathe.

> *I like nonsense, it wakes up the brain cells. Fantasy is a necessary ingredient in living; it's a way of looking at life through the wrong end of a telescope. Which is what I do, and that enables you to laugh at life's realities.*
>
> —Dr. Seuss

Tune In

I notice that some people seem to fear the word "meditation," thinking it takes great skill or is only useful if you are spiritually drawn, but that is simply not true. Meditation is for everyone, and as we become technologically advanced it is becoming even more necessary that we take time away from our gadgets and busy lives to be still with ourselves with no interference. I like to refer to meditation as "tuning in." Tuning in is exactly what it says: to tune in instead of tune out. Look inward instead of seeking outward. Tuning in or meditation is a practice to quiet and still the mind, resulting in a sense of clarity and peace. It's a time to connect and recharge.

Just twenty minutes of meditation a day has been shown, through research studies, to reduce stress, promote clarity, enhance creativity, promote work success, and improve your overall health and quality of life.

Once you have established this tuning in as part of your daily routine, you will begin to notice that your days become more productive, because with each moment of stillness, you attain more and more clarity. Think of it like a workout for your brain. Your brain needs a workout too, as it is a muscle, except you are pumping neurons instead of pumping iron, and keeping your brain strong is one of the best ways to counteract age-related loss of brain volume. After the age of thirty-five, we start losing brains cells at a rapid rate of one million per day. These brain cells are not replaced but meditation is known for helping to reduce this decline, as it changes the vibration of our entire makeup.

People who practice tuning in and meditating every day develop a magnetic, bright aura, one that emits a high vibration that others draw strength from.

HOW TO MEDITATE:

- Each day find some quiet time for yourself, free from others, electronic gadgets, or any other interferences. This is becoming even more important, as we all seem to be connected to our smartphones, causing our senses to feel overloaded.

- When you take this simple time for yourself, away from all the noise, you are able to hear your inner voice, but you have to be quiet enough in order to listen.

- When you *don't have time* to tune- n/meditate, is usually when you need it the most!

- Make a daily appointment with yourself as to when you are going to meditate. Honor the appointment with yourself just as you would any other appointment in your life. You wouldn't not show up to an important meeting, so show yourself the same respect.

- Start with five minutes and build up to twenty minutes per day. Set a timer so that you can actually tune in and not have to peak at a clock. Consistency is required to reap the full benefits and experience spiritual stillness.

The more you develop this practice into your lifestyle, the stronger your brain and intuition will become. Mental space opens up and you refrain from reacting impulsively and begin a more mindful, compassionate response.

When you are in the meditation state, it is similar to a deep sleep state. Time and space do not exist, only the conscious flow and connection to the divine. Thus, over time you will find that you require less sleep than someone who does not have a meditation practice.

Studies show that meditation can be especially effective for those suffering from anxiety or depression.

- Find a comfortable seated position, free from distractions and noise. Sit up tall creating length from your sit bones to the crown of your head. Either place your hands up or down on your legs. Up to receive energy and down for a more grounding energy.

- Close your eyes and begin to find awareness in your body by focusing on your breath. See where you may be holding onto any tension and on your exhale, let it go. Then begin a steady breath of inhales and exhales, trying to keep them equal in length.

- Lots of thoughts may come to mind. This is normal. Don't push them away. Let them come, acknowledge them, and let them go. As your practice develops, the thoughts will become less frequent.

It is also helpful to have a mantra (or a sacred sound) to come back to when the mind begins to wander. Sanskrit mantras are deliberately constructed so that they correspond with a particular type of energy. Serving as a vibratory link between you, your subtle body, and the divine.

Om (or AUM) is probably one of the most common and powerful sacred sounds and spiritual icon symbols. For many, Om is considered to be the first sound of creation. Having many translations, AUM is everything. It is the source, the vibration, and the consciousness of the entire universe.

Om is pronounced in three parts: ah / oh / mmm

You can also set an intention or repeat an affirmation that resonates with you. You can repeat one word, or a feeling that you want to attain, like gratitude, love, joy, or peace and synch it with your breath: for example, inhale love, exhale gratitude. This can be done silently in your head or you can begin aloud and then bring it inward after a couple of minutes.

One of my favorites, *Ra Ma Da Sa, Sa Say So Hung*, is a sacred healing mantra and is great for sending healing energy to yourself, your loved ones, and the world.

Meditation is only possible when all mental modifications (thought waves) have been stilled. This is completely subjective and only you are able to evaluate your progress.

> *Meditation is the art of breaking habits, to purify the mind and to take care of day-to-day things.*

> —YOGI BHAJAN

REFLECT

Set an appointment with yourself and respect it as you would any other appointment in your life and hold yourself accountable.

Describe your day in ten words then, after thirty days of tuning in (meditation), do it again and see for yourself.

_____

_____

_____

_____

_____

_____

_____

_____

_____

_____

_____

_____

_____

Live in Your Truth

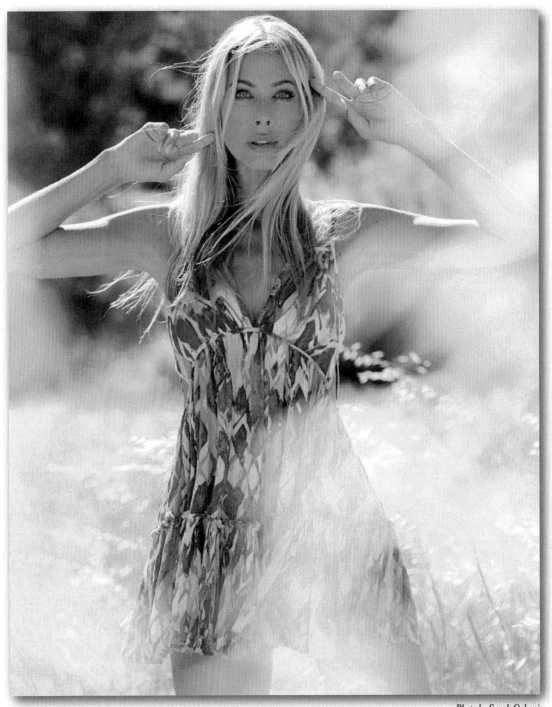

Live and speak from your heart and you will bring forth your true path and all the experiences necessary for your optimal life.

When you are living abundantly in your own truth, your body responds with optimal health and vitality. Allowing you to have a truly meaningful, purposeful life filled with contentment. This truth stems from your heart. When you allow your heart to carry you with the intention of living a truthful life, you bring your true authentic self forward.

Living your truth often requires you to move to a place of discomfort and unknown change. It requires that you move away from fear and limited beliefs and instead follow the yearn of your heart.

What gets us into trouble is when we allow our doubt and fear to creep in and run challenging scenarios and negative outcomes in our heads, which can actually bring those possibilities into reality. Living in fear creates illusions and roadblocks, disabling us from living our authentic true life. This is also true in our interactions with others. Fear of hurting others with the truth, so in order to avoid the hurt, we prolong the pain and tell them what we think they want to hear, completely abandoning our own truth and creating a false reality.

Lying destroys your credibility. When you lie, you are denying the other person an opportunity to make an informed decision because the information they are basing it on is false. Living in false character, or denying the truth, disempowers you and inhibits your growth and the growth of those around you. It creates ill thoughts in the mind that ultimately affects your health. When our words, thoughts, and actions are truthful we feel harmonious and are able to tune in to the consciousness that maintains our true self.

HOW TO LIVE IN YOUR TRUTH:

- Always speak the truth. Being honest and truthful in your communications allows the deepest, most fulfilling relationships and outcomes.

- Pause and be mindful of your tone. I believe that 90 percent of being successful at the other receiving your truth is in your delivery, not in the actual words you are saying.

- Ask yourself every day, "Where have I lived my truth today and where did I allow fear to take over?"

- Don't take what others say personally. Know that what others say has more to do with them than you. It is their truth not necessarily THE truth.

- Do not try to please everyone with your words. Be honest with yourself and avoid telling others what you think they want to hear. Not being honest prolongs the inevitable and could interfere with the best possible outcome.

- Have the courage to say no when needed. Have the courage to face the truth. This is living your life with integrity.

- Don't assume that people can't handle the truth. If you speak from your heart, those around you will be able to handle the truth and your conscience will be free of guilt. Speaking from your heart heals you and those around you.

- Trust yourself and trust your gut. Without trust, whether it's in friendship, family, or marriage, there is nothing to base the relationship on. Being 100 percent truthful and forthright with the ones you love is what builds trust in relationships.

- When there is fear and you find yourself in doubt, reroute your thoughts to your ideal outcome.

- Believe in your strength and your truth. Learn to trust yourself and have faith.

Our truth will set us free! We must strive to be more truthful in our lives, and when we do, the people who are meant to be in our lives will flourish because of it.

Of course there are scenarios where a *white lie* needs to be told. It is only in those rare cases where it is for the highest good, not a selfish act.

In Sanskrit, *satya* means actively expressing and being in harmony with the ultimate truth. In this state, we are aligned with our Knowingness.

Part 6
Connect

Have More Sex

We are all connected, to each other, to the earth, to the universe, to consciousness. When we truly understand that, we can begin to heal.

Connection is a primal need for humans. Touching, snuggling, caressing, and hugging are vital for us, enhancing our psychoneurological and immune function, helping us form strong emotional bonds, and uplifting our mood. During sex we are connecting skin to skin, enhancing the positive effects of human contact, and allowing us to receive the most benefits from this sacred connection.

When I say "have more sex," of course I'm not encouraging random sex with multiple partners. I'm talking about monogamous relationships where sex is already a healthy part of your relationship. I am also talking about pleasuring yourself!

I believe "the good stuff" is the actual orgasm. Orgasms release hormones, such as oxytocin, a hormone that can make you happy and less stressed. But even if you don't have an orgasm, you will still reap plenty of benefits.

For example, sex can help to keep you fit because having sex for thirty minutes is equivalent to fifteen minutes of working out on a treadmill.

Sex can also prevent common ailments because during an orgasm when oxytocin is released, it increases your pain threshold. So no more headache excuses. Sex just might be the cure for that throbbing in your head, along with soothing your nerves, and easing menstrual cramps and joint pain.

Not motivated yet to have more sex? Well that can be because you aren't doing it enough! Having sex will make sex better by improving your libido. The more you engage in sex, the better your libido gets.

FOR THE GODDESSES:
Many women are not aware that the vagina is a collapsed muscle and just like any other muscle in the body, it needs to be worked out in order to maintain its strength, shape, and health.

Doing Kegel exercises on a regular basis can positively affect your sex life, remove stress, prevent incontinence, and increase vaginal lubrication and elasticity.

KEGEL EXERCISE:

1. First locate your pelvic floor area.

2. Then imagine trying to stop the flow of urine.

3. Once you have found your pelvic floor, tighten it for four seconds and then release it for four seconds.

4. Repeat this several times a day, gradually increasing to ten- to fifteen-second intervals of contraction and relaxation.

For the more adventurous, you can incorporate a *yoni* (sacred place) or a jade egg (a tool for awakening sexual energy) into your feminine workout. The healing jade egg gemstone is designed for women who want to improve their vaginal strength and to heal and harmonize with the most sacred part of their body. Eggs have been used in Eastern cultures for centuries and have a wide range of benefits. Some benefits include helping to prevent incontinence, increasing the flow of sexual hormones, increasing lubrication, heightening orgasms, and feeling centered and grounded.

Sex is a natural, organic, and vital part of all living things.

Get Grounded

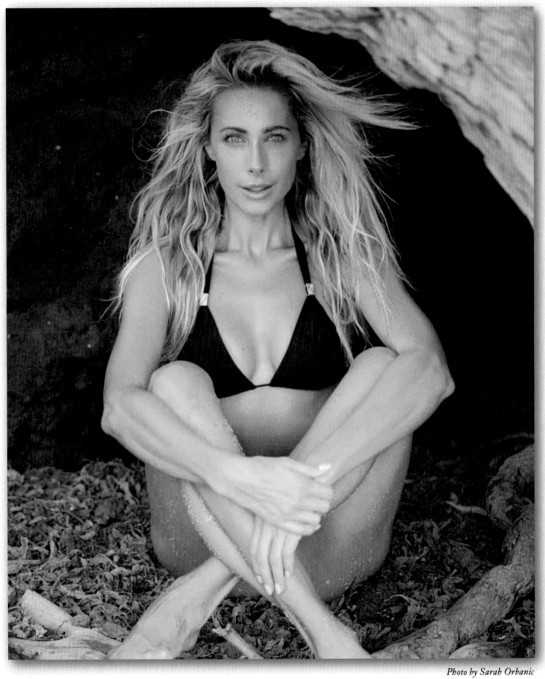

Photo by Sarah Orbanic

To be grounded means that you are deeply rooted and connected to your own spirit. Allowing you to be present, confident, healthy, and whole. On the other hand, when you are not grounded in your body, you can lack focus and suffer from fear, anxiety, and other health issues.

HERE ARE SOME WAYS TO MAKE SURE YOUR FEET ARE FIRMLY PLANTED ON THE GROUND:

EARTHING
Take your shoes off! Whenever you have the opportunity, let your feet touch the earth. If you are able to, lie down in the grass or in the sand or in the snow! Give all your troubles to Mother Earth and be open to receive her healing benefits. The next time there are not enough chairs, sit on the floor and ground yourself.

A daily practice of "earthing" can help you release any negativity and empower you on your path.

INTENTION
Upon waking, write down in a journal or recite them aloud your intentions (what you plan to do or achieve) for the day. This daily ritual helps you to gain more clarity for your day ahead, grounding you in your goals, assisting you in being more productive, and intentionally creating the life you want to have.

In the morning, say three things you are grateful for before your feet hit the floor.

BELLY TIME
Try sleeping on your stomach, like a baby! If you are a parent, then you have heard of "tummy time." Adequate tummy time is an important part of developing proper gross motor skills as an infant. It is also the beginning of learning how to root to the Earth, helping us to develop our brain, back, and neck muscles.

There is something very grounding about laying with your body facing down. To prevent kinking your neck, don't use a pillow when you do this. Sleep on your stomach in moderation, and when you do, I suggest wearing a satin or silk eye mask to prevent eye wrinkles.

YOGA
Yoga is a practice "through the self to the self." Yoga has the ability to positively affect all areas of your life. The lessons learned on the mat translate off the mat. Yoga is a tool to

create balance and harmony in your life. The asanas (poses) in yoga are based on the principle of "rooting in order to rebound." In essence, whatever body part makes contact with the floor presses down and roots itself to lift the rest of the body up, creating stability. As in life, you cannot succeed in anything without a firm foundation.

TUNING IN / MEDITATION

If the idea of sitting still with your own mind in silence sounds daunting to you then it is a sure sign that you will benefit most from doing so. It is absolutely the best way to ground, center and attain clarity for your life. The body benefits from movement but the mind benefits from stillness.

CRYSTALS AND ROCKS

One of the simplest ways to ground yourself is to put a crystal or rock in your pocket. This practice is especially great for kids. Every crystal carries a different vibrational energy that can heal, awaken, and ground an individual. Each person responds to certain crystals differently, and I believe it is best to let your instinct guide you toward what crystals you need in your life at any given time. Choose the crystals that you gravitate toward; that is, let them chose you!

When the roots are deep, there is no reason to fear the winds.

—*African Proverb*

REFLECT

Write three intentions that you want to create in your life. Feel the emotion of having already received them and trust that the universe will deliver.

_____

_____

_____

_____

_____

_____

_____

_____

_____

_____

_____

_____

Mother Earth

Our very being depends on us taking care of Mother Earth.

We live in a "throw away" society where our priority has become convenience for us but at the cost of our environment, which if we don't start taking care of is going to become a real inconvenience. Do your part and know that every person doing a little makes a whole. Share your knowledge with friends and family.

HERE ARE TWENTY WAYS YOU CAN BECOME MORE ENVIRONMENTALLY CONSCIOUS AND LOWER YOUR CARBON FOOTPRINT:

1. Reduce and reuse before you recycle and refuse to bring wasteful items into your home in the first place. Simply buying less stuff is the best route to lower emissions.

2. When you do need to make purchases, buy durable goods that last. Stop buying cheap, disposable items. Organize your office to switch to reusable dishes, utensils, and cups instead of disposables.

3. Eat fewer animal products. Most of us don't make this connection but the global livestock industry produces more greenhouse gas emissions than all cars, planes, trains, and ships combined.

4. Compost your food scraps, or you can throw all organic foods in the green bin. A lot of people do not know this but organic scraps can be put into the green bin, which is the bin where grass and leaves go.

5. Buy minimally packaged goods. For example, buy one large recyclable bottle of apple juice instead of a twenty-four-pack of individual juice boxes.

6. Bring your own canvas bags when you go shopping and not just for the grocery store, any store. Most states are finally banning plastic bags. Plastic bags end up in our oceans and pollute the environment.

7. Save the water. Turn the water off in between brushing your teeth, washing your face, shaving, and body scrubbing. Never leave the water carelessly running. If you

are waiting for it to warm up, then place a bucket underneath and collect the water to use for plants or animals. Nothing should be wasted.

8. Only wash full loads of laundry and wash clothes in cold or warm water, not hot. The same goes for the dishwasher. Only run the dishwasher when it's full and open the door for it to dry on its own, instead of using extra energy to dry it.

9. Unplug your gadgets and appliances when you are not using them, such as your phone charger, blender, toaster, hair dryer, and coffee machine.

10. Turn off lights. Be mindful and turn off unnecessary lighting.

11. Choose energy-efficient home and kitchen appliances.

12. Walk, bike, use public transportation, and carpool to run errands or get to work.

13. Drive an electric or plug-in vehicle.

14. Replace standard lightbulbs with energy-efficient lightbulbs. One bulb can reduce thirteen hundred pounds of carbon dioxide pollution during its lifetime.

15. Eat organic when you can. Choosing organic is the best for you and Mother Earth. Organic food is grown without synthetic fertilizers that pollute the environment.

16. Buy local as often as possible and support local businesses and farmer's markets.

17. Donate and support environmental organizations like Green Peace and NRDC The Natural Resources Defense Council.

18. Filter tap water. Do not support bottled water. It is not good for you and it is awful for the environment. Most of the plastic bottles end up in our oceans, fish eat the plastic, and then we eat the fish filled with plastic toxins. Get a good water filter and bottle it yourself.

19. Support clothing companies that produce responsibly by using sustainable methods and recycled materials.

20. Invest in your own source of renewable energy with solar, wind, and hydro power.

Give Back

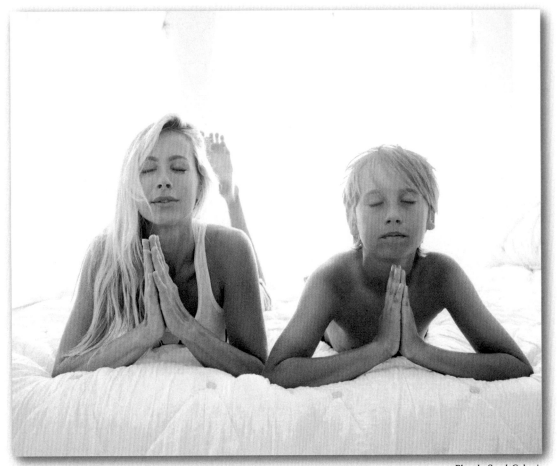

Photo by Sarah Orbanic

Y ou may be thinking, what does giving back have to do with my health? I believe that giving back can affect your mental state and your mental state affects your overall well-being.

I believe "looking past your own eyelashes" and helping others in need is one of the best ways to change your perspective and find gratitude in what you have.

By helping others, you in turn help yourself. Studies show that people who perform volunteer work or help those less fortunate have a greater zest for life and, in turn, are happier and healthier. You don't have to be part of an organization or a specific volunteer group, just helping others in time of need or making someone feel special is enough to make you feel good. The energy you put out into the world *does* matter. Every act of love and kindness raises the vibration of the entire universe. Small acts, when multiplied by millions of people, are what transform the world. It's the power of the collective. I believe that the best way to find yourself is to lose yourself in the service of others. When you give, you actually get.

Sometimes just lending an ear, a smile, or a hug is enough to be of help to another. When you know you have been a help to someone, it just makes you feel good. Whether helping others is a distraction from dwelling on your own issues or it is joyful, either way, your immune system reaps the benefits and thanks you.

HOW TO GIVE BACK:

- Get involved with a volunteer group in your community. Find something you are passionate about: the environment, animals, the elderly, children, or people less fortunate than you. If you don't want to join a volunteer group, then choose to be of service for your friends, coworkers, family, or people you see on a regular basis.

- Support a charity that you are passionate about and donate your time and/or money.

- Make an effort to help others even when it is the last thing you want to do. I believe one of our greatest tests is when we are able to bless someone else while we are going through our own storm.

- Pray for others, as much as you pray for yourself. We are all on this planet together.

Seva means doing a service, a service with no return. That is how grace gets multiplied, when you are not seeking any return.

—*Yogi Bhajan*

Signs That You Are Aligned

1. Stronger sense of compassion for all living things.

2. Loss of fear and a sense of calm.

3. Loss of judgment toward others and yourself.

4. Easily adaptable to all the ebbs and flows of life.

5. Making healthier food and lifestyle choices.

6. Rapid manifestation of intention.

7. Mission to be of service to others.

8. Power to create the reality you desire.

Part 7
Conclusion

Healthy Self
Heal thy Self

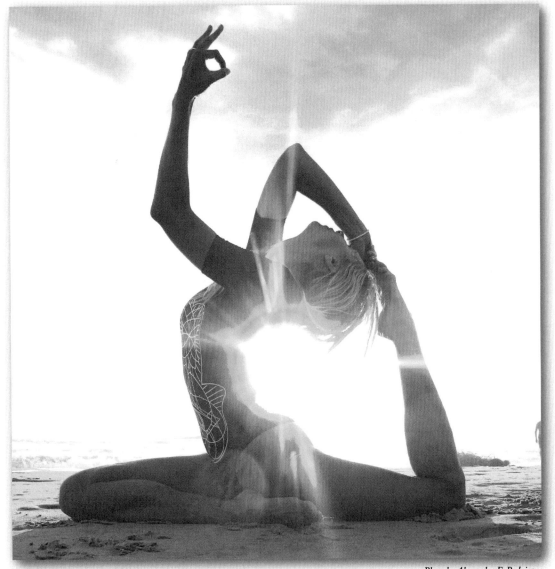

Photo by Alexander F. Rodriguez

The wound is how the light gets in.

- RUMI

You Have the Power

To grow and heal takes devotion and courage. It takes a willingness to be uncomfortable, a strength to open up old wounds that have been holding you back, a fluidity of mind to let the healing unfold as it desires, and a feeling of worthiness that you deserve the best.

And maybe it's also about unbecoming and unlearning things about yourself that are no longer working. A complete embrace of all the ebbs and flows of yourself and your life.

Take one day at a time, and with each moment, each breath, and each positive choice you make, you will begin to bloom and flourish more than you ever imagined.

When a flower doesn't bloom, you fix the environment in which it grows, not the flower.

You are not broken. You do not need to be fixed. You are perfect just as you are, but be tenacious in your commitment for a better quality of life.

Be patient, be kind, be prosperous, be radiant, be superb and *Be Golden!*

A grateful heart, followed by wise choices and persistence are the Golden Secrets to Optimal Health.

Bibliography

Balch, Phyllis A. 2003. *Prescription for Dietary Wellness*. New York: Avery Books.

Christensen, Kyle D. 2000. *Herbal First Aid and Health Care: Medicine for a New Millennium*. Twin Lakes, WI: Lotus Press.

D'Adamo, Dr. Peter J., and Catherine Whitney. 1996. *Eat Right 4 Your Type*. New York: Penguin Group.

Fischer-Rizzo, Susanne. 1990. *Complete Aromatherapy Handbook*. New York: Sterling Publishing Co.

Golan, Dr. Ralph. 1995. *Optimal Wellness*. New York: Ballantine Books.

Gottlieb, Bill. 2002. *Alternative Cures: The Most Effective Natural Home Remedies for 160 Health Problems*. Emmaus, PA: Rodale Books.

Hendler, Dr. Sheldon Saul, and David M. Rorvik. 2008. *PDR for Nutritional Supplements*. 2nd ed. Montvale, NJ: Physicians' Desk Reference Inc.

Hay, Louise L. 1999. *You Can Heal Your Life*. Carlsbad, CA: Hay House Inc.

Iyengar, B.K.S. 1979. *Light on Yoga*. New York: Schocken Books.

Iyengar, B.K.S., John J. Evans, and Douglas Abrams. 2005. *Light on Life: The Yoga Journey to Wholeness, Inner Peace, and Ultimate Freedom*. Emmaus, PA: Rodale Books.

Jensen, Dr. Bernard. 2000. *Dr. Jensen's Guide to Body Chemistry & Nutrition*. Lincolnwood, IL: Keats Publishing.

Kushi, Michio, and Stephen Blauer. 2004. *The Macrobiotic Way*. New York: Avery Books.

Lepore, Donald. 1985. *The Ultimate Healing System Course Manual*. Salt Lake City, UT: Woodland Publishing Inc.

Lockie, Dr. Andrew, and Dr. Nicola Geddes. 1995. *The Complete Guide to Homeopathy*. New York: DK Publishing.

Magaziner, Allan, Linda Bonvie, and Anthony Zolezzi. 2003. *Chemical-Free Kids: How to Safeguard Your Child's Diet and Environment*. New York: Kensington Publishing Corp.

Pizzorno, Joseph E., Jr., Michael T. Murray, and Herb Joiner-Bey. 2002. *The Clinician's Handbook of Natural Medicine*. St. Louis: Churchill Livingstone Elsevier.

Satchidananda, Sri Swami. 2007. *The Yoga Sutras of Patanjali*. Yogaville, VA: Integral Yoga Publications.

Sivananda Yoga Vedanta Centre. 1996. *Yoga Mind and Body*. New York: Dorling Kindersley.

Stein, Diane. 1997. *All Women Are Healers*. Freedom, CA: Crossing Press.

Weatherby, Dicken, and Scott Ferguson. 2002. *Blood Chemistry and CBC Analysis*. Jacksonville, OR: Bear Mountain Publishing.

WEBSITE SOURCES
American Heart Association. "Alcohol and Heart Health." Last modified January 12, 2015. http://www.heart.org/HEARTORG/HealthyLiving/HealthyEating/Nutrition/Alcohol-and-Heart-Health_UCM_305173_Article.jsp#.WJqHJoXFz2w.

Centers for Disease Control and Prevention. "Rheumatoid Arthritis (RA)" Last modified July 22, 2016
https://www.cdc.gov/arthritis/basics/rheumatoid.htm.

Food and Agriculture Organization of the United Nations. "Livestock a Major Threat to Environment." Last modified November 29, 2006. http://www.fao.org/Newsroom/en/news/2006/1000448/index.html.

Coconut Research Center. "Coconut (Cocos Nucifers) The Tree of Life" Last modified 2015. http://www.coconutresearchcenter.org.

Natural Health News Report. "Top 10 Reasons To have Sex Tonight" Dr. William S. Gruss. Last modified March 25, 2015. http://www.naturalhealthnewsreport.com/page/nhn/articles/healthnews/2015-03-25-116.html.

Harvard T. H. Chan School of Public Health. "Impact of Fluoride on Neurological Development in Children." Last modified July 25, 2012. https://www.hsph.harvard.edu/news/features/fluoride-childrens-health-grandjean-choi/.

Australian Broadcasting Corporation. "Coconut Water as Blood Plasma Alternative?" Karl S. Kruszelnicki. Last modified December 9, 2014. http://www.abc.net.au/science/articles/2014/12/09/4143229.htm.

Mercola.com. "Current Health News." Dr. Joseph Mercola. Last modified February 8, 2017. http://articles.mercola.com.

National Cancer Institute. http://www.cancer.gov.

People for the Ethical Treatment of Animals. http://www.peta.org.

United States Consumer Product Safety Commission. "The Inside Story: A Guide to Indoor Air Quality." https://www.cpsc.gov/safety-education/safety-guides/home/the-inside-story-a-guide-to-indoor-air-quality.

About the Author

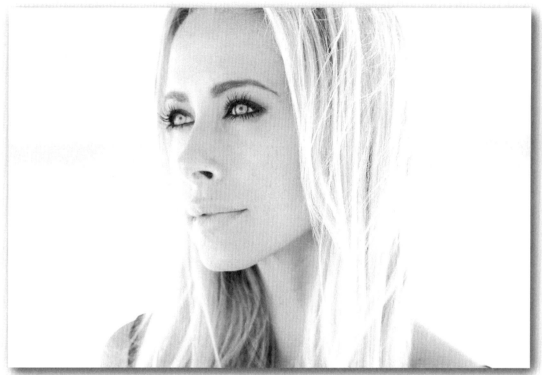

Photo by Ashley Noelle

Devoted mother, model, hatha-yoga teacher, holistic health practitioner, and creator of *The Golden Secrets*, Jesse Golden has used her multifaceted career as a platform to inspire and empower people all over the world.

Jesse's accomplishments began as a child when she became a ballerina in her mother's dance studio. Later, after putting the debilitating disease rheumatoid arthritis into remission through natural methods, Jesse has established herself as the face of hope in the health and fitness industry. She continues to thrive despite her diagnosis.

Not having the ability to answer all the e-mails and calls she receives from people asking for help, Jesse started *The Golden Secrets* to share the tools and tips that she has acquired, both from her journey back to health and through her life experiences. Jesse believes that every challenge we encounter is an opportunity for us to create more light for ourselves and for our world. *The Golden Secrets* is about health, beauty, fitness, parenting, spirituality, elevating consciousness, and empowering you to find your own path to fulfillment and optimal wellness.

This book specifically reveals Jesse's "golden secrets" to obtaining optimal health. Jesse believes that knowledge is power and that we need to take responsibility for our own health—for ourselves, our family, and the environment.

Stay connected via @jessegolden, @thegoldensecrets, and www.thegoldensecrets.com.

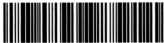

82918003R00113

Made in the USA
Lexington, KY
08 March 2018